Miracles in the Making

REV. DR. GEORGE S. BIEBER

Miracles in the Making

The Odyssey of a Healer

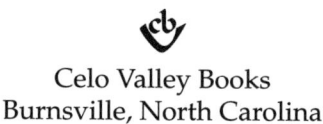

Celo Valley Books
Burnsville, North Carolina

Copies of *Miracles in the Making* may be purchased by sending
$15.95 + $3.00 shipping/handling to:
Rev. Dr. George Bieber
9 Westview Street
Grafton, MA 01519
georgebieber@aol.com

*All quotes from the Bible are paraphrases by the author
unless otherwise noted.*

ISBN 0-923687-59-9
Library of Congress Catalog Card Number 2001092705

Copyright © 2001 by George S. Bieber
All rights reserved.
Printed in the United States of America

No part of this book may be reproduced or transmitted in any form or by any means, electronic or mechanical, including photocopying, recording, or by any information storage and retrieval system, without the written permission of the publisher, except where permitted by law. Reviewers may quote if they give the title, author, and publisher of this work in the article or review.

To my wife, Montene, who is truly my angel

Contents

PART I: **HEALING FOR ALL**

The Gift 3
   Ways to View the Bible 7
The Calls 11
The Healing Ministry Begins 15
The Healing Ministry Grows 19
Questions on Effectiveness 25

PART II: **GROWTH**

The Gospel According to Edith 31
The Boy Preacher 37
   Juniata 38
   Clearville Charge 39
   My First Funeral 43
   Tatesville 45

Seminary and a New Desire 47
    Seminary (1943–1946). 47
    Boston/Mapleville (1944–1947) 48
    New Desires 49
    East Hartford (1947–1951) 51
Military Ministries. 53
    Geneva, New York (1951–1953) 53
    Iwo Jima (1953–1954) 59
    Morocco (1959–1961) 66
Civilian Ministries 71
    Martha's Vineyard (1961–1966) 71
    Marshfield (1966–1973) 74
        The Barn 78
        Walking Alone? 82
    Glastonbury (1974–1982) 86
    Spencer (1982–1988) 91

PART III: WHOM GOD EMPOWERS

Responding to the Call 101
Questions and Answers About Spiritual Healing 107
What I Have Learned About Spiritual Healing 121
Some Obstacles to Healing 127
    A Lack of Love of Self 127
    A View of Illness as a Result of Inadequate Prayer . 135
    A View of Illness as Punishment 136

A Death Wish	136
A Misinterpretation of Phantom Pain	145
Fears of Clergy	147
Unenlightened Church Teachings	152
Examples of Healing	159
AFTERWORD	169

APPENDIX: SOME THEOLOGICAL THOUGHTS

The Holy Spirit	173
Prayer	175
Sin	177
Frantic Fatalists vs. Kingdom Builders	178
Satan	181
Sermonizing	182
One Spiritual Adventure Group	185

PART I

Healing for All

The Gift

A driver brought them to my house. I had received a phone call from Rita, a woman who had been relieved of a cancerous tumor at a public healing service I'd held four years before. She had only recently learned of my new residence, and asked if she could bring some friends—a married couple—to see me.

I watched them as they parked. It took fifteen minutes for the man to get out of the car and into our living room. He was in great distress and bent forward with crippling arthritis. He had two arm canes. Rita introduced him as Henry.

His wife, Alice, Rita said, had Alzheimer's. I couldn't help but notice the frozen smile on her face. When I tried to talk to her the other two kept answering my questions. It was clear that they were accustomed to talking for her. I asked them to be quiet and persisted with Alice. She finally managed to tell me her name, but that was all. She settled back lethargically when I started to see what it was Rita needed.

Rita said she had developed some vision problems; she kept seeing lines wherever she looked. She also had shooting pains in her legs, but she'd had no recurrence of the cancer God had cured her of. I went to her.

"Stand up, please," I said. And when she did, I laid my hands on her head and asked God for healing. Within a few seconds I felt her relax beneath my hands, and I eased her down onto the sofa. She sat there for a while, overcome by the sensation of the healing.

Henry was sitting across from her, in a big armchair. I went to him next and helped him stand. He propped himself up with the steel canes. I put my hands on his head and prayed aloud for God to heal him. As he slumped down into his chair, the canes were dislodged from his arms. He remained still with his eyes closed.

I silently waited two or three minutes while Rita and Henry recovered from their healings. Then on impulse I went over to Alice and sat on a stool in front of her. Her eyes were alert now, and she was looking first at her husband and then across to Rita, both of whom were still motionless. I asked, "Alice, do you know what's going on here?"

"Of course," she said. "They have both been healed! Rita can see now and there is no pain in her legs. Henry will be able to walk."

"And what about you, Alice?"

"There's nothing wrong with me," she said. She began chatting about her family and named her children. She conversed with me as though she had been waiting to do this for some time. Obviously the Spirit was working: I had not prayed with Alice at all.

Now Rita "awoke" and discovered Alice talking with me. She watched and listened.

Next Henry was with us. He said, "I have to go to the bathroom."

"Go ahead," I said, "it's down the hall."

From long habit he reached for his canes. I moved them out of his way and said, "Stand erect, Henry," and he did! He walked purposefully down the hall and then returned.

When they went back to the car shortly afterward, Rita was carrying Henry's canes as he walked steadily and confidently. They left, a happy threesome.

• • •

I have been part of this kind of scene countless times in the past sixteen years, a scene of God at work through some person He has chosen as the conduit of His healing miracles. I am one such person, and I have experienced how persistent is the love of God toward His children. What follows is the story of how I came to have this gift to give God's healing, and the story of my own religious beliefs that have grown because of this gift. I want to tell my readers of spiritual healing as I have lived it, not as others speak of it. Most of all, I want to show how much God loves them; how anxious He is to heal them.

I want to testify to this: The healings I have been part of have taken place at God's initiative. Not one of us deserves to be healed. There are clearly no prerequisites for any given level of goodness or of faith on the part of the one healed. The prerequisites seem to be for other qualities entirely. And these prerequisites are sometimes difficult for "good Christians" to fulfill.

For this reason, I am concerned about the obstacles that, across the years, the Christian church has unwittingly placed in the way of healing. I say this as a dedicated United Methodist minister who is retired after serving sixty-four years.

It is not my intention to harshly criticize the church that I have loved and served, but to make some observations from my experience so that this situation may be understood and changed. It has been my experience that, indeed, God is love: His love is personal and overwhelming in its fullness. And it has been my experience that many "good Christians" are conditioned, through some interpretations of Christian teaching, to believe they are not worthy of the love God yearns to give each one of them.

God wants to heal more people, and He wants to make more people spiritual healers. Why, then, doesn't He? In my experience the reason lies in an ill person's own inability to receive His gift or in a would-be healer's lack of courage.

I will explain how I came to this belief by relating parts of my life story, including healings I have been privileged to be part of, and by interpreting some Bible passages in ways that my experience leaves me no choice to see in any other way.

WAYS TO VIEW THE BIBLE

It should be noted that what appear on these pages to be direct quotations from the Bible are not meant to be such. I believe the authors of the Bible were people inspired by God to write, and thus preserve, their God-given messages. Through much of my ministry I have found that Bible study helps people understand what God is saying to them if its method grows as those who study it grow.

I have to admit that some of the Bible says very little of relevance to me. The book of Leviticus is one such part, with its chapters on laws concerning offerings, sacrifices, the rituals after a healing of leprosy, and so forth. I do not get too thrilled with the various genealogies, either. (I especially started disliking them after someone prevailed upon us Biebers to have the family studied. Each family paid a portion of the cost, and when the book was published, I disliked it enough to suggest we pay a fee to have the whole thing hushed up!)

Most of the Bible, though, must be studied seriously.

To teach the Bible in the lower grades of church school, I have found that Bible stories, the life of Christ, and His teachings are best learned when taught as *fact* and then enforced with the words "Because the Bible says so." Questioning in this age group occurs mainly about *what* happened, not about what it *means.* In adolescence, teens ask questions about the relevance of the material. When they inquire about the value of the material to them, their questions should be discussed freely.

When adults study Scripture, I form what I call Christian Adventure Groups, so they can experience what Scripture has to say to them. I have found that these groups increase people's capacity to receive inspiration from the Holy Spirit. In this inductive method, which is described more fully in the Appendix, group members let go of extraneous details and give their ideas on what the passage means. All ideas are accepted equally. As members of the group see the passage's meaning develop, excitement grows—as it always does when the Spirit goes to work.

After reading Robert MacAfee Brown's *The Bible Speaks to You,* I decided that such inspiration is what is supposed to come from reading the Bible. Thus I have never regarded myself as much of a Scripture quoter. Each Bible passage ought to be interpreted in the light of our understanding of the whole drama—the whole of Scripture. For example, the idea of God outlined in the early books of the Old Testament can be contrasted with the picture of the loving God and Father introduced by Jesus. I find very exciting the drama of how our understanding of God developed over thousands of years.

So I claim the right to interpret a verse or a passage with the perspective of one who views the Word as a divine document that unfolds over time. For it is obvious that man's view of God is not all that changed as the Book developed; God's relationship with mankind changed as well. A reverence for the Bible is heightened by this approach to reading it. Word-by-word enthrallment robs us of a spiritually mature view.

It's an old story, but I retell it here to emphasize the point: A man took his Bible every morning and opened it at random to get his marching orders for the day. One day his finger caught the phrase, "And Judas went out and hanged himself." This was a little too much to take, so he tried again. This time the message was, "Go and do thou likewise."

I hope to encourage you to employ this inductive method in your own Bible study, and for this reason, throughout the pages of *Miracles in the Making*, I paraphrase biblical verses and give their source rather than choose one approved translation and give it verbatim. Such inspiration leads, I hope, to a closer personal relationship to God and a deeper prayer life.

Prayer and faithfulness to my own relationship with God have been an essential part of my life. I received the gift of spiritual healing that is illustrated on the opening pages of this book after forty years of asking God for that gift. When He gave me this gift, He did so suddenly and unmistakably. It is sometimes a struggle to correlate the certainty of my experience of God's healing with traditional interpretations of Scripture. Perhaps this is why so many mystics (of which I am not one!) were (and are) so often in trouble with the churches of their day.

I hope *Miracles in the Making* will lead you to a deeper understanding of what God desires for you. I hope it will give you confidence to ask Him for healing in your life. I hope it leads you to a deeper life of service to Him Who is Love.

The Calls

My call to the ministry was sudden, unexpected, and dramatic. I was attending a morning service at our home church, Third Street Methodist Church in Williamsport, Pennsylvania, and the preacher that day was a retired minister who had once served that church. He spoke about service to God. He mentioned the long list of pastors that the Methodist conference had sent this church over the past twenty years and said, "But this church has never given one person back, to serve God as a minister." I was twelve years old. Usually I spent the time during the sermon gazing at the organ pipes high above the pulpit. (As I stared at them they would melt together and even today I don't know how many there were.) But this time I was listening, and I was propelled from my seat. I walked down the aisle and got the preacher's attention (and that of my stunned family) by announcing, "I'll be the first."

My family took me seriously, and from that day on I began preparing myself to be a minister. On the occasion of my thirteenth birthday my mother gave me a small, portable Communion set with my name embossed in gold—but misspelled. I still use it. The next year I got a funeral manual!

At some juncture in my teens my mother told me of the circumstances of my birth. She regarded it as a miracle or at least an event that portended my future. My father, with my older brother and sister, had gone to church. My mother was alone at home. She heard the church bells ringing when I decided to be born. It was Christmas Day. When the family came home my mother showed them the new addition to the family. She told them that she had given me over to God's service, and she just *knew* I was going to be a clergyman. Despite her certainty, however, my mother never tried to influence my career choice. She waited until after I signified my intention to be a minister before she told me the story.

• • •

The call to the gift of healing at age sixty-four was just as dramatic. I had prepared myself through educational channels to be a minister and a psychologist. It had been my dream to be chosen by God to be a healer. The apostle Paul spoke of gifts given to chosen persons. One of them was the gift of healing. I had been for many years a pastor and a counselor. I had sought to help people as best as I could in those roles. I found myself inadequate, however, to meet the deep needs of God's people or even to show them the wideness of God's love. In response, I sought the gift of healing, not because I wanted to feel special, but because I felt that the gift of healing was needed in the world.

I began praying for this gift nearly forty years before I received it. And yet when it came, I cannot say I expected it.

I was alone, browsing through the Scriptures to see if there was any special inspiration for me that day. A passage I had read many times before came into view. In the fifth chapter of James, the writer was speaking of going to an elder of the church when you are sick and having the elder lay hands upon you for healing. Suddenly I was shaking with emotion. This was it! I had received the gift! It was certain!

At that time I was the sixty-four-year-old pastor of the United Methodist church in Spencer, Massachusetts. It was 1985. Without consulting anyone I put a small announcement in the church bulletin for the following Sunday. It simply said, "The pastor is available for anointing for healing." No one asked me to explain that note, but the next day I received four phone calls. Two were for minor ailments, two for cancerous tumors. I went to all four homes, laid my hands upon the afflicted persons, and asked God to heal them.

The two with minor ailments were healed instantly. The other two felt a strange warmth coursing through their bodies from my hands. Both men were facing operations later that week and both decided to have further testing. When their CAT scans showed that the tumors had shrunk, the operations were called off. Several weeks later additional tests came up completely negative. No cancerous tumors could be found.

We were astounded at the power of God that was so obviously at work in these people through my hands and prayers. For whatever reason, God had certainly gifted me with a responsibility equally as sacred as my calling to the ministry.

I thanked God for that gift, and promised to use it in His name. Nothing was now more important for me than to continue to follow God's will. I would be a conduit of His healing.

That was true in 1985, and it is still true today, over sixteen years later.

The Healing Ministry Begins

I decided to hold a healing service immediately. I called a priest friend of mine to see if he knew of a format for such a service. He did not. So I made up an order of service and met with my church's lay leader and its organist. A healing service was announced in the bulletin for the very next Sunday evening.

Curiosity brought some people, loyalty to their pastor brought others. We had a sizable congregation that very first time—January 1985. We used a form for the service that I had long envisioned during the years I had been praying to become a spiritual healer. That same form is still used today.

We sang some hymns, discussed some Scripture verses concerning healing, spent some time praying for people whose names had been submitted for prayer by those who attended. Then I gave a talk on healing and explained the laying-on-of-hands process. I made the statement that I would heal no one; God would heal through me. The people then formed a line and came to the altar area. Each person told me what his or her need was, and I placed my hands upon him or her and prayed that God would heal this person, offering myself as God's instrument of healing.

I remember well the feeling of aloneness, of terror, which I felt when I walked up into the altar area alone, prayed at the altar, and held my hands high before the central cross. As I walked down the steps and waited for people to come forward, it seemed like an eternity before anyone came. The organist was playing softly. Where would I go if no one came? I wondered in panic. No trapdoor was available.

My terror was for naught. Today I am sure that it was my ability to accept that terror, to be ready for ridicule should I get in God's way, that allowed me to receive His gift of healing in the first place.

I was told later that, within a few seconds of the call the seekers formed a line that reached to the front door. From the parishioners' viewpoint, there stood a man waiting to help heal them. There was nothing tentative about their response. Instead there was almost an epidemic of expectancy. And as people began to witness miracles at the front of their church, they rejoiced, and shouted, "Praise the Lord."

God healed many that day. We decided to hold a healing service each month.

After the second monthly service one of the members of the church, Joyce Freeman, wrote a description of that healing service as she experienced it. It said in part:

A couple of hours before the service it began to snow. George began to worry about the older people coming. Or who would come. He was anxious for it to begin, and paced back and forth. As I went into the sanctuary there were people scattered about the church. Our own people, and strangers. More came.

There was an aura about the whole room. George sang and then we all sang hymns. Then he spoke on healing. A calm, confident talk. Then he made a call for healing and asked those who wanted God's healing to come up front. We sang two stanzas of "Just as I Am." No one moved. He just stood there. As we began singing the third stanza, it started. One by one they came and stood in a single line. It was unbelievable. It seemed after a while that the line was endless. People in the background sang quietly while the healing took place. George gave to each individually, keeping some longer than others. It was sad yet beautiful. It seems we all afterwards were amazed. No one wanted to leave. We were quietly loving one another. God's amazing grace.

Now I will attempt to describe the most intense part of the service. The actual healing power. One person at a time, he would put hands on the head of that person and pray. I could see the intensity in his face. I could feel it. It was like a jolt. Then he would put his hands on their shoulders to steady them. Some would barely be able to stand. George's face would take on a different appearance with each one. I don't mean his face changed. I mean you would see him relating personally, individually, with each one. As he let go of one he would take hold of another (and not just literally). One of the men of the church would help people who were so shaken that they needed help getting back to a seat. Miracles were happening.

The Healing Ministry Grows

From this beginning a team was formed, a format for the service itself was defined, and healing services were scheduled for the first Sunday of each month. Local newspapers were generous in their news coverage, printing personal interviews and notices of meetings. Several of my closest ministerial friends invited us to hold services in their churches. No official recognition from United Methodist hierarchy was received, but as more and more miraculous cures took place, the attendance improved by word of mouth. I soon found it necessary to also meet with individuals in my office for prayer and for the laying on of hands. I did not charge for this healing ministry.

I began to compile a book of affidavits but abandoned this practice because of a reluctance to cause embarrassment for the persons involved, and also because I didn't feel a need to prove the authenticity of spiritual healing. I denied permission for a Boston TV station to bring cameras into the sanctuary and record the healing line. Jesus Himself constantly tried to ward off the acclamations of those He healed. I wanted to do likewise.

• • •

The healing team, then and today, consists of a song leader and general overseer of the program, ushers, soloists, and assistants to stand near me while I pray healing prayers over each individual who comes forward. These assistants are needed because many who feel a healing taking place are temporarily weakened. Rather than allow them to fall to the floor, the assistants step forward to help the healed. This assistance allows an atmosphere of reverence to be maintained, rather than one of unwanted hysteria due to healed people falling to the floor because of momentary weakness or fainting.

Special music is offered for each service. The soloist(s) and the song leader lead these hymns. The program overseer then greets the people and makes a few announcements. Specially chosen Scripture verses have been distributed by ushers to several people. These are read and I comment on their meaning. Then I stand by the altar rail. I try to relax the people by telling them how the service will develop and by offering a prayer.

I amplify the Scripture readings, pointing out how clear are the messages that God wants His people to get well, and be well. He stands ready to bring healing, I remind them.

A leader reads the names on the prayer request slips, and

I ask God to bring healing to those persons. The request slips are then entered on a printed prayer list so that I can pray for them each day at home.

Next, I explain how people should form a line if they want to come for individual healing. I go back to the altar for my own silent prayer, and then step forward to receive the people. If there are persons unable to come to me, I go to them.

The congregation sings hymns or listens to music so that no one can hear a petitioner's request. I listen to each person's need, then lay my hands on the person's head and ask God to heal him or her. At least two assistants are beside me, in case this person needs help back to a seat.

The service is ended when the line is finished. We join hands and sing a song of thanksgiving, and I offer a benediction.

• • •

God is all-good. He does not inflict illness on His people. He can do anything and heal any disease. I am one of His agents, and my long experience of being part of miraculous restorations enables me to affirm that no case coming to me for Him to heal is hopeless. There is no such thing as terminal illness in God's parlance. I know that He is anxious to restore. The only requirement to receive His healing is to be open to that healing power. It is my strong faith in healing that enables me to seek the removal of any blocks between the one requesting and the God Who is giving healing out of His grace through Jesus Christ.

I have seen cancerous tumors disappear, and crippled legs and withered arms grow strong. I have seen people wake from long-term comas. I have seen spiritual wholeness attained and broken relationships mended. I have seen sight and hearing restored. I have seen mental illness, arthritis, leukemia, Alzheimer's disease, emphysema, psoriasis cured. . . . The list of cures is long.

• • •

I remember a young man who had an eye injury from a piece of fireworks at a local Fourth of July display. He proceeded to institute a lawsuit against the town.

He came for healing and the sight of his injured left eye was restored. He canceled the suit.

• • •

A high school principal faced bypass surgery for at least one clogged artery. He came to me with respect but skepticism. He could not accept spiritual healing intellectually. But like many others, he was willing try anything.

I laid my hands on him and prayed. I then asked him to request more testing before he submitted to surgery.

He called me a few days later, crying, almost incoherent with joy. "I have had more tests and there are no blocked arteries!" he said.

• • •

Two sisters came to my office in Spencer. Each had been diagnosed as having a cancerous tumor of the brain. I prayed with each, laying my hands on each of their heads. I felt the power surging from me to them. God was at work! When I finished, they sat quietly for a short while and then asked me what they could expect. Would the tumors shrink? How long would it take? Did I think the prayer had been successful?

I told them, with the bravado God charged me to have, that their tumors had disappeared. Further tests proved this to be the case.

• • •

I can almost always tell when a person has arthritis just by touching the person's shoulder. Then my hand goes to the affected spot and I pray. The relief is instant. God is great and God is good!

• • •

A woman named Martha had her hearing markedly improved. She began to bring her friends to me. One day she brought a woman named Joan to my office, introduced us, and left the room. I talked to Joan about healing.

She was embarrassed to be there. Nothing in her Christian outlook included healing and she had heard some wild tales about the subject. She stood, though, and I laid hands on her lower back where her arthritis was making her life miserable.

Afterward, I could see that she had been profoundly affected. I eased her back into her armchair, where she sat with her eyes closed. But Joan's two arms were being held straight out!

I called Martha back into the room, and she looked curiously at her friend sitting there without moving, her eyes closed and her arms held out. Finally she called out, "Joan! Joan!"

Joan opened her eyes.

"Why are you sitting there with your arms held out?" Martha asked.

Joan looked at her arms and found that she could not lower them.

I went over to her, grasped her arms, and they fell into her lap. I wondered if God had been playing a little trick on us.

The arthritis was gone, whatever the arm position may have meant. Two weeks later Joan came to see me with someone else who needed healing.

Questions on Effectiveness

I don't keep score, but my estimate of instances of success for healing is 80 percent. I have kept in touch with a great many people who have been cured, and not once has any of them regressed to the ailment they sought help for.

What of the other 20 percent?

Sometimes, when I have been asked to pray for healing for a person—even some people I am personally attached to—I am given the message that there will be no physical cure for this one. When the disease not healed is an imminently fatal one I exercise compassion for those who will soon leave this earth and also for those who grieve the impending loss. I remind them that this life is not the end for God's faithful servants, it is the beginning of a more glorious life. I remind them, too, that they will meet again in the heavenly realm. When the disease is degenerative, and will lead to eventual death, I remind the person that they will be sustained to meet the suffering with God's help. Sometimes we pray together, often with the person's doctor, for a painless passing.

These reminders that God sometimes refuses to heal a

person (for reasons we may not understand) are particularly poignant to me as I complete the writing of these pages. I am currently seventy-nine years old and ill with emphysema. I have been told that God does not want to give me healing. I don't know when I will be called to go to Him, but I do know that it will be sometime not too far in the future.

Finally, there are people whom God would cure if they were able to receive His healing. These are the people who trouble me the most. Not because the failure is their fault, but because we churchpeople have failed them. I do not believe that religious faith on the part of ill persons is a prerequisite for them to be healed. Or even that there needs to be a "middleman" between God and those in need of healing. It does seem, though, from my experience, that ill persons must believe that they are *personally* worthy of healing. I have seen how anxious God is to heal them, how tremendously God loves them—not because they are "good enough," but just because they are His children. God loves each of us so much that, indeed, if we were the only one on this planet, He would still want to heal us. This is the simple yet difficult-to-comprehend concept of grace. I will speak of it further.

As I have aged, I have often wondered why God answered my prayers and gave *me* the gift of spiritual healing. Certainly the gift is just that—a gift—and not something I "earned." Certainly others have prayed for such a gift for just as long a time. Is the answer simply that God often chooses unlikely persons to hear His specific calls? Or is there something in addition to that, something in my life that "qualified" me? I have concluded that, perhaps, the way I was led to respond to God's inspirations was more than something that made me seem unusual to others. Those responses also helped me develop some qualities necessary for one who is ready to pass on God's healing to His children. I offer some of these incidents as food for thought.

PART II

Growth

The Gospel According to Edith

I was brought up in the church from babyhood. The Bieber family—my brother, Charles; my sister, Mae; and Mother and Dad—attended regularly. My mother directed hymn-singing from our rear pew (though this was not her assignment); she loved to sing and could always be heard. Dad had a deep bass voice with only two or three notes, but he sang as though he had been trained.

Though our church had a succession of ministers who seemed to come and go so quickly that I hardly got to know their names, the people of the church were faithful. The church survived and even thrived because of their efforts. I progressed faithfully through the various departments of the Sunday school. Though I was not very well-behaved, I learned the Bible from a series of dedicated lay teachers.

I still remember those wonderful teachers. The one I liked best was Clyde Wurster. He worked as a mechanic and his hands were rough and blackened from changing car batteries. His breath smelled richly of pipe tobacco. He was always prepared for the lesson and provided his own interpretation of the Bible stories. He made the heroes of the Old Testament live: David, Samson, Daniel, Joshua, and the like.

I remember a sermon by my father's brother Edmund, a pastor at another church, when I was eleven years old. He called it "The Gospel According to You," and it was a message that affected me for the rest of my life. In it he said there was a fifth gospel in addition to the ones written by Matthew, Mark, Luke, and John. That was the one written by "You"! We were to interpret the Good News from the Bible according to our understanding of the words and themes, and by using the Holy Spirit as our guide. I found this approach exciting!

My mother, Edith, also had her own homespun theology, and it affected me deeply. It was a system of beliefs that the Spirit led her to find relevant. She taught that gospel of hers to her children by word and by example. She did not expound on concepts like the Trinity, she told us how to relate to the different persons of God. God was the Creator and Father, and the Holy Spirit was God within us—within everyone, that is, though not acknowledged and recognized by many.

When she spoke of Jesus she meant the Son who walked about on earth and taught and healed and preached and led a group of disciples. When she spoke of Christ, she meant the one who was (and is) our Savior and Lord. This distinction in her wording helped us to always know which aspect she was talking about.

Mother also taught by example and by her homespun wisdom. Behind our house and next to the railroad track was a gathering place for bums. These were the Depression days, and among those so-called bums were men of social standing who had fallen upon hard times and who were traveling about looking for work. Stokers on the locomotives that pulled the freight trains past that spot were "careless" with their shovels and threw some coal along the tracks for those traveling men who had dropped from a boxcar when the train had slowed for a curve. The men would gather around a fire and share what food they had. We three children were not allowed to visit them, but they would visit us. They would come knocking at our kitchen door and Mother would bring them in. Dad would come home from work expecting, perhaps, beef stew and it would be gone. We would have cornmeal mush, warm pie with milk, or broken pieces of my mother's home-baked bread with sugar and milk. Dad never complained about this, and I cannot remember that any of us children did either.

Some of our friends were hard hit by the Depression. Dad had a job managing a laundry, and Mother took in boarders. We always had a big garden, so our cellar shelves were full of home-canned vegetables, chicken, and pork. On the day when people went downtown to get their dole of surplus food, Mother would sit on the front-porch swing and greet them as they passed by. As they returned with their wagons and baby buggies, she would come out and express admiration at what they had received. Would they be willing to trade some of the pepper, cornmeal, flour, sugar, for things she had on hand? They would! We had a vast supply of those surplus food items, too, in the cellar.

Once, we children came racing into the house to tell her that a family of Wops was moving into the neighborhood. She knew the word, and told us not to use it or any other derogatory term. She gathered us around and reminded us that our beloved uncle Harry was an Italian, and that our great-grandfather was Jewish.

On another occasion the neighborhood kids used the *n*-word for a new family on the block and implied that we didn't want "that kind" of people near. Mother told us, "Don't you remember that your father worked for a black man when he worked at the Aulston family laundry? The Aulstons had a son born right after you, George, and I nursed both of you—white you and black James Aulston—because Mrs. Aulston was unable."

Each week we were given a nickel to put in the church offering plate. I could buy a lot of jujubes with a nickel. I asked Mother, why did I have to give so much to the church? Where did the money go? She reminded us that the money was carried forward and put on the altar. It was still there when we went home. "After the service," she said, "angels come and take that money and give it to God."

Company took top priority in our house. They were served first at table. They could freely use our toys. It was expected for the three of us to sleep on the floor while our cousins occupied our beds.

The day before Thanksgiving we were put at the table and required to list twenty-five things we were thankful for.

At the beginning of Lent we had to volunteer three things we would give up for that penitential season.

On Good Friday we spent an hour at the same table in silence, thinking about our Jesus on the cross.

Across the years I have come to realize how valuable was this training and how effective was my mother's style of planting good Christian ethics in her children. It is her examples of putting Christ's teachings into practice that I have tried to follow in my own life and in my ministries.

The Boy Preacher

In 1937, at age sixteen, I met with members of the Committee on Ministerial Standing, who grilled me on my knowledge of Scripture and on the validity of my calling, and then required me to give an impromptu sermon on one of the subjects they assigned on the spot. I apparently did well, for I thereby earned a local preacher's license.

A retired minister in my hometown of Williamsport, Pennsylvania (he had once been pastor at Third Street Church, where I answered the call when I was twelve) asked me to help him with two rural churches. He was frequently ill and unable to lead worship, so I began preaching and leading worship on a regular basis. Until I was more confident in doing this I asked my family and friends to stay away!

I found that the people of those churches were intrigued with having a boy as their preacher and they were very supportive of my attempts to follow God's call. For a time I wrote a column entitled "From the Boy Preacher" for our weekly newspaper.

After high school I attended a junior college in my hometown, so I was able to continue preaching, this time as pastor of another rural church. I stayed with them two years until I was ready for a four-year college.

I hoped to go to Juniata College, in Huntingdon, Pennsylvania, for my B.A. I asked the superintendent of that Methodist district if there were any student charges in the area. He was happy to suggest the Clearville Charge in Bedford County; Juniata College was just sixty miles away from the parsonage. I was assigned there in 1941, and I served while I attended Juniata.

JUNIATA

Juniata College is a college with direct ties to the Church of the Brethren. The Church of the Brethren is an offshoot of the Mennonite Church, a sort of modern version that permits electricity, telephones, automobiles, and so forth.

My brother Charles had graduated from Juniata and had joined the Brethren, eventually becoming ordained as a minister in their church. (He and his wife, Mary Beth, went on to spend fourteen years in Nigeria in the mission field, where the emphasis was on providing schooling and medical care for the Nigerians. After he returned from Africa he held several churches and eventually became Moderator of the denomination. Even after retirement he spent five years as pastor of their largest church in the quaintly named town of Ephrata, in the middle of the Pennsylvania Dutch country.)

My own experience in the Juniata community was not as smooth as Charles's. I was not aspiring to be a minister like some of my classmates; I was one already—a cause of some jealousy. I did not feel called to join the Brethren either, so my Methodism set me apart. And because of the demands of my pastoral schedule I was away weekends, so I was unable to participate in most of the social activities of the college.

Moreover, I did not have a very keen interest in a lasting romance with any of the Brethren girls, not even Mary Beth's sister. These young women were eligible, but my focus was on my drive to finish schooling, so I made a poor suitor.

I was at Juniata for classes and little more. Years later I attended a class reunion and discovered that very few even remembered that I had been in their class!

CLEARVILLE CHARGE

There were five churches on Pennsylvania's Bedford County circuit: Shreves, Pleasant Union, Stevens' Chapel, Robinsonville, and Clearville (where the parsonage was). I was scheduled to preach three times each Sunday on a rotating schedule and lead the adult class at each church where time permitted.

There was a large parsonage in Clearville, which was a small village of some twenty homes, in farm country.

I well remember driving down the two-lane macadam road from Everett into Clearville that first Friday. I had a twelve-year-old Chrysler Club coupe that I'd bought with the help of a finance company (original cost sixty dollars; final cost, ninety three). It served me well. When I arrived, I found a general store, parked in front, and went inside. A number of men were sitting on benches chewing and spitting tobacco into buckets. They all became quiet when they saw me enter. By their standards I was well dressed. I wondered, at first, if their silence meant they were hostile to preachers, but I soon learned they were only curious. My arrival was expected, they told me respectfully.

I asked the store owner for a can of beans and a loaf of bread. He gave me the beans but said I'd have to get the bread from Mrs. Hann, the woman who lived across the road from the parsonage.

The white well-kept Methodist church was next door. I moved the car there and went into the parsonage, feeling as though a hundred eyes were watching. I felt more like that when I went outside to the bathroom, which was a two-holer in the backyard! I used the water pump just outside the kitchen door to wash up.

After I unloaded my clothes, I looked through the house. It

was clean and furnished, and the rooms were large. Three bedrooms were upstairs; downstairs there was a living room, a dining room, and a big kitchen with a stove that burned either oil or wood. I preferred wood and there was some left for me in a box. The cellar held a large wood-burning furnace.

Next I went across the street and asked to buy some bread. The dear old widow lady asked me in and we became acquainted. She introduced me to her adopted daughter, Frances, who was my age. I was asked to stay for supper but told them I was already getting my supper ready.

Back in the parsonage kitchen I could find no can opener and no large knife. I found a pair of pliers in the car and managed to open the beans. I was about to rip chunks from the still-warm bread when I heard a knock on the door. There was the daughter, Frances, with my meal on a tray—all laid out on plates with silverware! I tried to hide my beans but she just said, "Enjoy your supper," and went back home.

After I got settled and made the bed in the room above the kitchen, I went across the street to return the dishes and express my thanks. Before long Frances was playing the piano and we were all singing. I learned that the Hanns went to another church in the village, Clearville Christian Church.

According to my schedule of services, Pleasant Union Church, which had a sizable congregation, was to be my first service. That first Sunday went well. Then it was on to

Robinsonville, which wasn't a village at all. Lots of wagons and a few horses were tied up outside the church. I led the worship and taught the class that followed. As I walked out the door, a family stepped forward and invited me to lunch with them. I gladly went along and we had fried chicken. (Every week I went to someone's house to eat those Sunday meals and we almost always ate chicken, or occasionally canned pork tenderloin. The larger farm owners would also invite me to fill up with gas at their tank.) The third service of the day was at Stevens' Chapel, where we sang "Beulah Land" each Sunday because it was the only hymn the pianist could play. After another Sunday school class, I was free for the day. Then it was back to Clearville to load my car, secure the house, and say goodbye to my new friends, after which I still had to drive sixty miles back to Huntingdon, where my roommates waited for me. If I was "flush," we went to Skip's for a soda and a doughnut.

The Methodist district superintendent had not told me what my salary was. I soon learned that whatever came into the offering plate was what the preacher was paid. I earned approximately one hundred dollars a year from each church.

The people of those one-room churches and chapels were grateful to have someone serve them. I had been duly appointed by the Central Pennsylvania Conference of the Methodist Church to be their pastor, and they showed no particular surprise at my age. They gave me no special treatment, nor did they remind me of my inexperience. Though I had no idea that one day I would be given the call to be a healer as well as a minister, I was finding out that following God's call at such an young age as mine was not as difficult as it might seem. I did have one moment of puzzlement, though.

In Clearville, one Sunday, I walked down the aisle of the full church to begin the service. Before I got to the platform an elderly man reached out and gave me something. I announced the opening hymn, then looked to see what I had been given. A thin dime! Was this man telling me I was worth only ten cents to Clearville? I wondered uneasily. Then I put the dime in my empty pocket and decided that was a foolish thought. I was where I was meant to be, doing what God had asked me to do. The dime was most likely meant as a meaningful gift.

Just as my congregations seemed to accept me without question, my family and friends, and my college mates also, acted as if working as a pastor while going to school was nothing unusual. I did encounter some attitudes among my congregations, though, that were new to me.

MY FIRST FUNERAL

As was my custom, I stopped one February day at the general store and chatted briefly with the men on the benches and made a small purchase. The men had accepted me by now and everyone called me "Preacher George." On this day one of the men walked out with me, got rid of his cud, and asked me if I had time to do a funeral. I assured him that I would take the time! (My pastoral appointments allowed me to conduct funerals and weddings, but not baptisms and the Lord's Supper. An elder from Everett came periodically to take care of those matters.) "When do you want it and who is it?" He told me it was his uncle Jeb and there was no real hurry, he had died the week before. I pressed him to call his family together and have it done that week at his home. I made a special trip for it.

When I arrived, it was a very cold day. All the men were in the living room, gathered around the potbellied stove. The women were cooking and chatting in the kitchen. I waited as long as I could and finally ventured, "Where's Uncle Jeb?" They pointed to an adjoining room. There was no heat in that room and Uncle Jeb was lying on a cot wrapped in a sheet.

I called the assemblage together, marched them into that room, and read the service from Mother's old gift, my funeral manual. Next, Jeb had to be buried.

Unceremoniously, one man took hold of Jeb's head and another took his feet. They carried the frozen form out behind the barn, where they had dug a hole. I read the committal words and Jeb was rolled into the hole, naked without his sheet. No undertaker. No death certificate. No fanfare, and no mourning that I could see. To them, the funeral was mainly an opportunity for the family to get together. (I delight in telling this story to my funeral-director friends.)

TATESVILLE

My old Chrysler behaved well for me, but eventually it developed a leak in the radiator. I put cans of junk in it to fill the holes, and it smelled bad but still dripped. So I gathered a few water jugs, filled them up at school, and set out for my churches. I estimated that I could go about sixteen miles before the car got hot and I had to add water. I soon had a system of fill-ups at farmers' wells along the way. That way I could make the trip. When the weather grew cold, however, the radiator froze and cracked the engine block. I managed to get it to my uncle's garage and he bought it from me, trading it in for a 1929 Ford Model A. I learned later that he welded the block, cut out the rear seats of my car, and drove it as a truck for several years!

Once, while I was still driving the Chrysler, I miscalculated the amount of water I needed and drove down a short street in a village called Tatesville. My car and I were steaming, and a man came out and offered water. While he filled the radiator I walked down the road, where I had spied a church just like the five I already had.

The man filling my radiator saw my interest and told me it was Methodist. The minister from Everett had come out to serve the people until he had tired of this three years before, he said. The church had been closed ever since.

I asked him if he thought there would be people interested in having it open again, and he assured me that the church was missed. After introducing myself, I told him I'd be back.

I clearly felt that God wanted this church reopened, so the next Monday I drove from Juniata to Tatesville and began to make calls. That very next Sunday we started services again. The people in the area had cleaned the sanctuary and gathered their hymnals from their homes and were all set to go. So I added a fourth service to my Sunday schedule—this one on Sunday evening.

Within a few months Tatesville clearly was a success, so I notified the district superintendent. Tatesville was formally added to my appointment, and it grew to have the largest attendance and largest budget of any of the six churches I served.

Seminary and a New Desire

SEMINARY (1943–1946)

After graduation from college and sad farewells to the people of my six churches, I went to Boston to attend Boston University's School of Theology. I chose BU because Methodists preferred their ministers to be graduates of BU, there were a number of student charges available nearby, and because I had a full scholarship there. I augmented my scholarship by washing dishes in an upscale restaurant four days a week—for one dollar each mealtime and my choice from the menu for meals, which I ate in the kitchen.

I was thrilled at the stature of the professors at BU, whose theology school at that time was on Mount Vernon Street. Below BU was the exclusive Louisburg Square, where some of our theologues earned money reading to residents.

I had a good background in the Bible and found the courses easy. Homiletics (the art of preaching) was fun, too. I had already had several years' experience in that area.

In addition to working toward my S.T.B. (Bachelor of

Sacred Theology) at BU's three-year seminary, I intended to get a doctorate in pastoral psychology, but I soon changed that secondary degree to one in clinical psychology. The latter degree program offered more variety in courses for credit, and as a clinical psychologist, I would be able to work in the field of physical and mental therapy as well as in the church. To this end, in addition to the seminary program, I took graduate courses both at BU and, thanks to an agreement between the schools, across the river at Harvard. By the time I finished at seminary in 1946, I had almost a year's accumulation of hours for future use toward my Ph.D. in clinical psychology.

BOSTON/MAPLEVILLE (1944–1947)

While I studied, I also continued as a preacher. After several months in Boston, I accepted an appointment to the Mapleville/Glendale Charge in nearby Rhode Island. These two communities were more than 90 percent Roman Catholic, but the small Methodist communities were fervent. The Mapleville church was unique: It had been built largely by mill owners who modeled it after a miniature cathedral. The Glendale church was several miles away, largely attended by various officers of the mills and their families.

Part of the week I stayed in Boston in housing provided for the theology students. My roommate was also a student pastor.

NEW DESIRES

One evening at a gathering in my room with two friends, we discussed the conditions of the student churches in the area of the school. For years the members of these small churches had been served by neophyte pastors who spent two years with them and then moved on to greener fields. I wondered aloud what would happen if some men were to decide to stay longer and really apply themselves to church nurture and growth. We found ourselves praying about this and decided to take a vow to serve only small churches throughout our entire careers. "Small churches" was easy to define: We meant those churches that paid only the minimum salary set by the annual conference each year. That vow was kept by two of us: the one who spent his entire ministry in small churches on Cape Cod and me.

My vow would cause me trouble in the future, since a minister's prestige with a conference is often based on the size of the churches he or she has served. Hence, some of my views were summarily dismissed instead of being heard objectively. Instead of as one trying to remain faithful to his valid call, I was often seen as one breaking the rules, one who should simply be dismissed as a "maverick" (which I am, but I'd like to hear my views considered seriously). Still, I'm glad I did not choose to climb the ladder to the larger, better-paying churches with the nice parsonages. I don't regret that each time my district superintendent asked me to take a larger appointment, I quietly and persistently refused and subsequently told him of a struggling church I would like to go to instead. This vow eventually took me along a path that led to receiving the spiritual gift I began to seek while at BU.

• • •

The desire to ask God for the gift to heal came during a study of the epistles of Paul while in seminary. I was already deeply committed to the idea that the call to the ministry was from God and now I was fascinated by what Paul listed as special gifts in the twelfth chapter of First Corinthians. Among these special gifts was the gift of healing.

Coupled with this fascination was my dismay at the attitude I noticed among my fellow students, who regarded the many miracles performed by Jesus and recorded in the Gospels as an interesting array of biographical accounts of the great things Jesus did—and nothing more! I viewed the great things He did as more than part of a historical account: I viewed them as challenges to us to do the same, following in His footsteps.

I remembered how He once said, "The one who believes in [Him] will do greater things than these" (John 14:12). To think of doing miracles with a power given me by God produced in me an exciting, all-encompassing feeling of hope that someday I would be anointed to be a healer in addition to being anointed as a minister. I began to pray for this gift of spiritual healing. The year was 1945.

Like my fellow seminary students in 1945, many clergy today are reluctant to accept the validity of the gift of healing because they carelessly restrict the possibility of healing to that done in the lifetime of Jesus Christ and His apostles. To them, it is difficult to believe that such miracles could occur today. I have always been saddened by this conclusion.

• • •

While at BU and while serving in Glendale and Mapleville, Rhode Island, I married Peggy Work, a Methodist I'd long known from my hometown of Williamsport, Pennsylvania, who proved to be a great asset to my ministry. She played the piano, organ, and accordion and was beloved by the people on the charge. On the days when I was in Boston, she remained in the parsonage at Mapleville.

EAST HARTFORD (1947–1951)

The year after my graduation from seminary in 1946, an older student asked me to accept an appointment he was leaving in East Hartford, Connecticut. This was arranged, and in 1947 I found the small church at the end of a dead-end street. It was largely unknown in the community. I dug into the work with passion.

I called on every house in a widening circle and concentrated on several government-sponsored "villages" within the town. The attention shown these people was richly rewarded. At the end of the first six months we doubled our membership.

During those years I also taught in the local high school as a full-time substitute, teaching various subjects every day and doing my best to be more than a baby-sitter.

While in East Hartford, I managed to continue my studies, taking courses at Harvard and also traveling down to North Carolina, to study at Duke (parapsychology) and at the University of North Carolina. These courses helped me farther along the road to getting my clinical psychology doctorate.

I left East Hartford to fulfill another dream. The church I had served there had begun plans for a new church in another location, and this was accomplished within two years of my departure in 1951.

Military Ministries

GENEVA, NEW YORK (1951–1953)

I had long wanted to enter the United States Air Force as a chaplain. I had been too young to be considered as a chaplain during World War II, but now, with my divinity credentials from Boston University, I was accepted into the military as a chaplain in 1951.

After Chaplains' School at Fort Slocum, New York, I was sent to the mammoth basic training center outside Geneva, New York. Peggy and I had a daughter, Becky, by then and had found housing on the base. Soon after arriving we were blessed with twins—Shirley and Susan—bringing the count to three daughters.

At Sampson Air Force Base I began work in one of the training groups, interviewing each incoming recruit, giving character guidance lectures, and listening to a long list of complaints from the green-fatigue-suited basic airmen.

I noted that no activities were provided for the large number of teens on the base. For these dependents of officers and noncoms there was only a bowling alley and the base theaters. So I sought space for a teen center. Soon I found a vacant building with an old sign on it: BASE MORGUE. No one I asked knew anything about it.

I made my way inside and found it to be an ideal place. The hobby shop provided me with a sign that said SAMPSON TEEN CENTER, and I put it in place of the morgue sign. Various supply sergeants scrounged furniture for me. I posted notices around the base and the center was soon in business. A short time later an officer showed up and told me I had stolen his building! Too late for him—the commanding general's twin daughters were already active participants in the new teen center!

We had board games in the club, a soft drink dispenser, and a record player. We held parties and dances, but the major use of our building was as a hangout for the military's teens. Then we got the idea of going on trips. People at the motor pool could find regulations allowing them to bus us to places within a few miles of the base but not to Radio City Music Hall in New York. For that trip, we had to earn some money.

By some chance I learned that the Goff Salt Water Taffy factory was in Leroy, New York. I called them and then visited them. They were anxious to have groups sell their taffy. Each box, sold at one dollar apiece, would pay us fifty cents! I signed a contract, we loaded the pickup truck with cases of candy, and came back and unloaded it at our clubhouse. The kids were convinced their fathers could sell some at their places of work, and that their mothers could help, too. We started out that way but didn't even sell the truckload. So I came up with another plan.

We got more taffy, a lot more taffy, and began to visit the barracks at night. In my first lieutenant's uniform, accompanied by two boys carrying boxes of taffy, I would approach the CQ (the officer in charge of quarters) of a barracks. He would call his basic airmen to attention, and the boys would work their way down the line, selling taffy. Sales were brisk.

Then our girls found a way to sell effectively. They went to the base theaters when training films were scheduled to be shown. As the various flight groups marched in, in single file, our girls would stand at the door and offer the candy. It sold!

Goff's had to stay in operation an extra week that winter to provide us with candy, and the kids in the club headed for New York City in a commercial bus. All our expenses were paid from the profits of our sales.

It was decided to transfer me into the position of police and prison chaplain. In an office made for me in the stockade, I set to work interviewing and then counseling the prisoners. Most of them were jailed for noncriminal military offenses, though some were jailed for more serious offenses, such as assault upon a flight leader.

It became apparent that some of the Air Force enlistees at Sampson were not honestly trying to serve. But exactly what was going on was not clear. I made a file on each of these men and noted their behavior until I saw a pattern: Some of these miscreants had devised a system to get out of the service with a BCD (bad conduct discharge). To do this, they would go AWOL for two or three days, then get caught, tried, and sentenced to thirty days. Later they'd go AWOL again, and again be sentenced to thirty days. They'd go a third time, stay away for a week or two, then be given three months. After getting out of the stockade they would have to begin basic training all over again. Their next AWOL would last a month, and it would result in being given six months' jail time—and a BCD, which is what they had been bucking for.

Given the draft system at the time, this was unjust behavior. Accompanied by the stockade commander, I took my study, with the statistics I had compiled, to the commander of the base. In a few days the "reward" for this type of behavior was removed: All these men's BCDs were erased and the men started basic training again, this time with no BCD in the future. A small percentage spent their two years of contracted time in either basic or confinement!

The men this affected did not take my actions personally. They, like others, knew me to be a man who was firm but fair.

One of the problems I faced with the prisoners in the stockade was providing religious services for them. This issue had been avoided until I moved in. As a start, I decided to take them to an evening service conducted by a Southern Baptist chap named Livy Cope. He was a likeable fellow and had services with fiery sermons and a lot of singing. His church was within walking distance. I received permission from the CO and signed up the men to go the following Sunday.

To my utmost consternation, when I went to line up the churchgoers I found them being searched as they came out of the gate. Air Force police had lined up on either side of the column of men heading for church. At each end of the line were police pickup trucks holding men carrying shotguns. Guards on foot called cadence as my two hundred or so men marched to chapel.

When we arrived, we were told to sit together and cause no disturbance. The guards remained outside. After the service, the men were lined up again and marched back to the stockade.

I didn't go into the stockade that night. I was too embarrassed on their behalf.

I dreaded going to work the next morning, and when I did, I heard what I expected to hear: "Who wants to go to church like that?" "Everybody was driving by staring at us." "We felt like we were criminals." They concluded that they weren't going to chapel again.

I pleaded with the stockade commander to allow me to take them without guards. He refused: It was against regulations.

I confided my problem to the base commander and he gave me permission, reminding me that it would be my neck if anyone escaped.

I told the men the new plan, and they agreed to return to church the following Sunday. One of the bolder fellows told me it would be nice if they had something to put in the offering plate. Another asked if they could have a smoke break.

The next Sunday a few more volunteered for chapel. I gathered them outside the gate in a loose column and gave each man a cigarette and a dime— items I had been given by one of the Catholic chaplains. The prisoners lit up, and we were off in a cloud of smoke while the guards stared at us from behind the fence. During the service the men sang lustily and put their dimes in the plate rather proudly. (After the service we waited outside until Chaplain Cope's assistant brought me back the dimes, which we used the following week.) We never lost a man going to church. Not one attempted to escape.

Of the fourteen chaplains who came to Sampson from Chaplains' School, Livy Cope and I were the only ones promoted to captain eighteen months after our arrival. When I arrived at my next base overseas, I was awarded my first Commendation Medal, given to me with an impressive ceremony on the forsaken island of Iwo Jima. That medal was given for action outside the scope of regular duties, for my broader dedication to the task of chaplaincy.

This recognition of my effectiveness was important to me. But it had more meaning than I understood at the time. The person it acknowledged was a person who was learning to use whatever resources he could find to fill the needs of others—sometimes at the risk of his own reputation. In the following years I would become more practiced at taking a risk to fill need.

I believe it was this courage to face failure and ridicule that God needed in me before He could give me the gift of healing. The following stories illustrate some ways my nerve grew.

IWO JIMA (1953–1954)

With my wife and our three daughters housed in an apartment in our hometown of Williamsport, I flew to Japan. I had been assigned to the small airbase on the island of Iwo Jima. The purpose of the base was to maintain a landing strip for emergency landings and refueling. In the thirteen months I spent there, I saw no need for those tasks to be performed.

The Second World War and the terrible battle for this strategic piece of real estate located south of Japan had destroyed all vegetation. The landscape was covered with black rock, volcanic sand, cliffs around the beaches, and the remains of war: planes, tanks, trucks, jeeps, ships sunk offshore, pillboxes, huge guns, and man-made cave and tunnel openings.

Iwo, "the Black Pearl of the South Pacific" as we called it, had a military complement of about three hundred enlisted men and a few officers. There was no native population, there were no females, and there was no civilization. A few warehouses and some Quonset huts housed all the activities.

Morale among the U.S. troops there in 1953 was very low because no one had done anything to improve conditions on the island since the war. There was no recreation program, no entertainment, no sports, and no educational effort. Boredom was rampant: An alarming number of the men had gone "rock-happy" and been relocated to either Japan or the States.

Prior to my assignment there, the island had been served by a series of visits by various chaplains who would spend a week on temporary duty holding religious services. But with my background I was expected to do something about the morale problem during my appointed one-year tour.

The base commander, a pilot with his first command, was genial, soft-spoken Lieutenant Colonel Charles E. Dean. He cooperated in every way with the ambitious program I set up to give the men something to do.

I had nothing to work with, so I finagled a trip to a base in Japan, where I spent a couple of days scrounging equipment.

There too, the cooperation was superb. I found a vast array of supplies, including hundreds of books for a library, textbooks and courses for educational purposes, a flock of Japanese bicycles (which didn't hold up after the first race down the runway), sports equipment of all kinds (including ice skates, which we fed to the sharks!), and a complete radio station, which I found boxed and dusty in a warehouse.

It was like Christmas when I returned to Iwo with these finds. I assumed responsibility for all the equipment and began to establish a leisure-time activity program in which every man was expected to participate. Of these men, 167 had never graduated from high school. I enrolled them in evening classes and made attendance mandatory. Before they left, all but six received their GED. I taught the necessary courses and gave the tests.

I was able to do this, thanks to the University of Maryland. For a time, before coming to Iwo, I had taken some courses at the University of Texas. The University of Maryland accredited me to teach military personnel high school courses, and encouraged me to finish my degree so that I could teach college courses as well. They gave me credit for all the graduate courses I had taken since 1943, and I took correspondence courses in psychometrics through them. I then submitted a dissertation on military AWOL and retraining, and was finally given the long-sought Ph.D. in clinical psychology.

The men on Iwo who were high school graduates also needed intellectual stimulation. I required them to enroll in college courses. The course choices were criminology, American literature, and creative writing. I taught these courses too, using curricula from the University of Maryland. Through the university the men who successfully completed a course received three hours' credit for it.

Each man was ordered to write home once a week. I wrote sample letters for them to copy, and their names were crossed off when they satisfied the order.

Louis B. Mayer sent us crates of movies, which we showed two or three nights a week, using the side of one of our buildings for a screen. Morale began to improve on Iwo Jima.

• • •

All personnel were obliged to enter into some phase of the sports program I introduced. Softball, basketball, horseshoes, tennis, and boxing were the most popular. We formed teams; for example, the men of the motor pool played against those in food services. Eventually we began sending teams to tournaments in Japan, where our small base contended against bases with thousands of men to choose from.

We knew that our outfit, the 6415th Air Base Squadron, was presumptuous in competing with those large bases, but it gave us a chance to visit Japan for a few days and it helped alleviate the boredom on Iwo. We entered teams and accepted the fact that we never won. Then we became aware of a strange development: By studying, playing, and working together we had formed a familylike unit, one which we had not really consciously planned. People began to think, Why *can't* we win a trophy? We're getting tired of losing.

We heard of an upcoming boxing tournament and thought that could be our area of success. We chose three men and began training them. We set up a ring and sparred with them. We put them through a rigid course of physical training. The time came and I took our medic, a heavyweight, a light heavyweight, and a middleweight to Tachikawa.

Our heavyweight fought the first night we arrived and was knocked out before the end of the first round. The next night our light heavyweight lasted three rounds, by clinching and running from his opponent. The third night we found our middleweight on his dressing table, stone drunk from a bottle of saki. I had trained to fight in my teens, so I put on his equipment and entered the ring under his name.

I knocked my opponent out in the first round. The head chaplain of the Far East Air Force leaped into the ring and announced my identity. He had been surprised to see me, but he saw to it that I returned for the next fight. I knocked my opponent out on the fifth night, won, and became the middleweight boxing champion of the Far East Air Force! We returned to the Black Pearl with our first trophy.

Morale was at an all-time high in our Iwo family now. I hadn't planned to get quite so heavily involved in my own program, but I was not immune to that urge to see our crew win.

• • •

One of the things that brought a lot of "life" to the Iwo base was the communications equipment I had brought back from my first scavenging trip to Japan. The men were thrilled at the idea of having their own radio station, and various "experts" showed up to get it together and on the air. There was no thought of the Federal Communications Commission, or of permission from the Far East Network to go on the air. It took us several weeks, but one night we finally managed to figure out how to get on the air. Small radios were placed all around the base with the dials set on various settings, until we found the frequency we were broadcasting on. Lo and behold we had made it: We were live!

I became the officer in charge of the station, so I appointed a station manager. Together we began to set up programs. We had quiz shows pitting one base group against another. We played country-and-western music from old records. Our own Ron Newell took the name the "Black Pearl Plowboy," and his programs were popular. We had popular music and even some classical. We interviewed interesting people, and since we were the only ones on the island, we interviewed each other.

There was trouble when others found out that our signals were carrying too far and blanking out some stations in Japan. Finally a team came down and made adjustments and commissioned us as VOIJ, the Voice of Iwo Jima. We were now legitimate.

When I finally left the island I was invited up into the cockpit to hear a program of farewell music engineered and selected by Ron. Songs included were "So Long, It's Been Good to Know You" and "A Stranger in Paradise."

• • •

Although I managed to keep busy on Iwo by teaching school and giving GED tests, by running the library, by editing the weekly newspaper (*The Suribachi Sentinel*), by overseeing the radio station and sports activities and other odds and ends, I had plenty of time to think. I kept on praying that someday I would receive that gift of healing. It meant more to me with each succeeding milestone in my life.

• • •

In 1954 my assignment at Iwo Jima ended, and I returned to my family in the States. An example of how morale at Iwo changed in the year I was there can be seen in George Fuller. He was an airman who came in 1952 to spend a couple of months on temporary assignment on the Rock, doing his specialty: air installations. He liked being there so much that he asked if I could help him extend his tour with us, thus shortening the time he would have to spend in the Far East, away from his wife back in the States. I was able to pull some strings and he did stay with us.

Years later, in 1993, George worked for months to gather some of the men who had been on Iwo from 1952 to 1954. It was like gathering a lost family together, but he persisted. He found me after weeks of searching. We had a reunion in Florida that year and about forty of the Black Pearl vets gathered joyously for several days, sharing many stories of our adventures together on the Rock. The extent of the ties we had formed after the low-morale days of 1953 proved to be strong. We Black Pearl vets enjoyed being together those many years later. And since that first reunion, we have had four others, including even more men, along with their wives.

MOROCCO (1959–1961)

After a fulfilling five-year stint as base chaplain at a fighter base on Long Island (Westhampton Air Force Base) my family and I were shipped to Morocco. Here my efforts to expand the chaplain's program were thwarted for a time because the chaplain on hand outranked me by more time in grade. But I was promoted to major in 1960, and he was transferred to one of our bases in France. Then I organized the Nouasseur Teen Club for military dependent teenagers and a chapter of the United Protestant Fellowship, which met on Sunday evenings in a building we found unoccupied.

Peggy and I became close with an English missionary couple who had worked in Casablanca for more than thirty years. They had not made any converts but they energetically conducted a medical and dental clinic for some of the many Jews who lived in that large city.

Just as I thought we had things running smoothly, a major earthquake hit the town of Agadir. Several thousand people were killed, more were buried alive, and the city was laid to waste. In order to help, our base commander described the calamity through military channels and asked for permission to donate supplies from the scores of warehouses remaining from World War II. I knew it would take at least three months to clear the red tape, so I went ahead and commandeered a fleet of trucks, stocked them from the military's warehouses, and delivered the goods (amounting in value to at least a million dollars) to the stricken area.

I was put under house arrest and faced a general court martial for unauthorized use of government goods (in other words, larceny). But the world press told the story, and I was commended and given a humanitarian award by the Kingdom of Morocco. (Our base supply officer thought he faced a major problem writing off all we had appropriated until it was learned that no inventory of that war surplus existed.)

• • •

It was at this large airbase in North Africa that I was first used officially as both base chaplain and base psychologist. I had offices in the chapel and also at the large hospital. I went back and forth on a motor scooter.

Any cases of suspected malingering or of illness or disability whose source could not be determined by various tests were referred to me. I still had not received the gift of healing I was praying for. Each day I encountered situations where that gift would have been invaluable. My psychological background came in handy, though, and I used it as best I could. The commander of the hospital later officially commended me for returning to duty a number of airmen who had been hospitalized for strange infirmities.

One of these was an airman from Kentucky who trembled constantly in a state of terror. He was medicated, but his medication only took the edge off his hysteria. They brought him to me. I allowed him to sit quietly for a while as I made notes about my previous case interview. Finally, informally, I started to speak with him about his home folks and how he liked the military. He gradually grew more calm and finally burst out with his story.

He showed me a letter he had received from a former girlfriend in the hills of Kentucky. He had indicated to her that he was no longer interested in furthering their relationship and her anger had turned to vengeance. She told him in her letter that she had prevailed upon an aunt of hers to put a hex on him. This airman had been brought up in an area where hexes are a very real part of life, and her hex had filled him with terror.

Where in all my textbooks could I find a cure for this (or any) hex? I wondered.

Then an idea came to me—it didn't make scientific sense, but I thought it might prove effective. I solemnly opened my middle desk drawer and brought out various objects in my fist, which I opened before him as I mumbled unintelligible phrases. There was a cross, a Saint Christopher medal, a Mass card, and a small rock. Each was passed in front of his eyes as I mumbled in a monotone. Then I scrambled to my feet, rushed over to him, and clasped his head in my hands.

He slumped forward in his chair and, in a few moments, stood up and began walking around the room more calmly than before. I went to lunch with him and he was later discharged back to duty.

Clever psychology, or healing?

• • •

Another airman, a clerk in the orderly room, had a paralyzed right arm. He could not lower it and no one could pull it down. After a few moments of interrogation in a kindly fashion, I learned that two other clerks had been transferred out of the orderly room and their work piled on his desk.

I used a sympathetic tone as I quietly assured him that he could not be expected to do the work of three men and that he should relax. He said he would try. I said, "Let's shake on it." When he started to do so, his right arm came down. He went back to duty the next day.

Hysteria had paralyzed his arm, and given him an excuse for not being able to do the impossible amount of work assigned to him. I phoned his first sergeant and he solved the work situation.

My willingness to use unorthodox, but effective, means of psychological healing in that hospital office may well have been a kind of preparation for my later healing ministry.

Civilian Ministries

MARTHA'S VINEYARD (1961–1966)

I returned to civilian life in April of 1961 and notified my bishop's office that I was ready for appointment at the upcoming annual conference in June. Two weeks later I received a call from Mr. Stephen C. Luce, wealthy resident of Martha's Vineyard in Massachusetts, asking me to consider coming to his church in Vineyard Haven. He assured me that the salary would be open. I told him that I received my appointments from bishops and I took only the conference minimum salary. Two days later my bishop phoned and suggested that he wanted me to go to Vineyard Haven!

So to Vineyard Haven my family and I went. I also acted as pastor at Lambert's Cove, which was a small church near the eastern coast of the island. It had a small core congregation in the off-season. In the summer it was full of worshipers from various inns that had a tradition of sending their patrons to that quaint church a few miles away.

I loved the work on the island, especially after the summer

people left in September. I worked hard to build up my congregation, and we soon had a youth group of thirty-six, all of whom eventually joined the church together at a confirmation service that broke all records for attendance and membership gain.

• • •

A congregation of American Baptists in Oak Bluffs had a church called Bradley Church, which was attended by the African-American residents. They asked me to serve them because they couldn't afford to hire and house their own pastor. Their service was held on Sunday afternoons and lasted the usual hour except during the summer season when the cooks, maids, and butlers of the large estates came to be together. Some of those services lasted between two and three hours. I stayed with them for almost three years, until one Sunday two visiting gentlemen arose after the service and informed us that the American Baptist Convention had sold their building. That brought many tears, especially when we learned that a VFW had purchased it. A priest friend and I devised a service of desanctification of the sanctuary and of the altar furnishings, and people from all the island churches attended.

The good people of Bradley Church left an impression on me. Their faith was real. They were devout, they were loving, and they accepted me into their family. The meals we had in an adjoining room were not only sumptuous, they were soul-satisfying. I kidded them about a "prejudice" against me: They had color and I had none—I was just pale white. But I could do no wrong with them. When I revealed to them my dream of becoming a spiritual healer, their response was simply, "Keep on praying."

• • •

My pastorate on Martha's Vineyard was a delight. The church in Vineyard Haven grew strong. Our youth group made three bus trips off-island, all expenses paid with money we had earned. Most of the money was realized from variety shows held at the local high school. People from all over the island volunteered their amateur and professional talents. I acted as emcee and used my love of singing to contribute two lip-synching numbers, one as Eartha Kitt and the other as Teresa Brewer.

In my leisure time, my friend Ed Donald and I did a lot of fishing—with little luck. We would start out after supper, and go to a secluded spot on Vineyard Sound. There we would throw our lines out, weighted down with lead sinkers and baited with squid. Often we fought a fish up and down the beach only to discover we had caught a useless sand shark or a skate. Nothing to bring home. Sometimes an apparent failure is the beginning of something good, though. Despite the lack of catching food fish, I later found those memories of the sunset on the water, of the smell of salt, and of the companionship we shared had become lasting ones.

MARSHFIELD (1966–1973)

After five years on the Vineyard I found myself getting restless. I wanted more challenges. I had heard of the possibility of beginning a new United Methodist church in Marshfield, a rapidly growing town north of Plymouth on the South Shore. I drove up one day and learned that a small group was meeting in a beautiful old farmhouse on the main street through the town. I found one of the couples and stayed with them that night. I decided to ask to go there as a full-time minister.

Our three girls were in high school and Peggy elected to stay on Martha's Vineyard, working in a bank. The bishop appointed me to Marshfield, and my three daughters and I moved in. Furniture in our new home was sparse and we just "camped out" for a time. But it wasn't long until we had everything we needed.

Men of the small group busied themselves by converting a greenhouse connected to the main farmhouse into a rustic chapel that could seat about seventy-five. The downstairs of the farmhouse was converted into classrooms, and bathrooms were added. The upstairs made a comfortable home for the minister and his family. We had three bedrooms, a large living room, a bath, a kitchen, and a study. We named the church Marshfield Methodist Church.

Becky, my oldest daughter, finished high school, and then she was off to Deaconess Hospital nurses' training program. She completed the course and received her R.N. degree. A short while later she married a young man from a Vineyard family. Then the twins graduated from Marshfield High School. I taught there as a full-time substitute, mostly in math subjects, which were my worst subjects when I went to school. The church started to grow.

I made calls in an ever-widening circle around the church. The people responded and began joining our group. We added a second service and then a third during the evening hours. We started a building program and a building fund drive.

Though Marshfield Church owned fourteen acres in the middle of town, I dreamed of building our sanctuary on adjacent property at the top of a tree-topped hill. A wonderful widow, Mrs. Benjamin Ellis, owned that acreage, and when I called on her to tell her my dream, she served me tea and said she and her husband had vowed to keep that land, as it was a bit of old rural Marshfield in the middle of town. I was disappointed.

Two weeks later she phoned and asked me to come over. I had barely sat down when she said, "I have decided to let you have that land for your church if you take down only the trees necessary to drop a church in." Overjoyed, I asked what the price would be. Her answer was, "I'm going to give it to you. I believe in dreams too." Today the main hall of the church on top of that hill is named Ellis Hall.

We built our church in those woods. The department of architecture of the United Methodist Church sent plans for an all-purpose building. It featured one large room with a stage at one end that could hold the altar. Folding chairs would be used instead of pews, and we could hold fellowship and public suppers in the same area where we worshiped.

We wanted to build a finished church, though, feeling that if we used the model they offered we would never have anything better. To us the atmosphere of the proposed building would seem to indicate that we had failed to meet our goals from the very beginning. We found a corporation that had built several churches in New England, and we worked with their architect instead.

After getting the dimensions we needed for this type of building and an adjoining parking lot, I marked all the trees that would have be cut down. I used my ax to fell many of them and sold the wood for fireplaces. The finished building did appear to be "dropped in," just as Mrs. Ellis had envisioned. The trees that were still standing became a background for the floor-to-ceiling clear glass window behind the altar. We now had a beautiful one-story sanctuary with an adjoining office area, and a two-story wing that housed a large hall, a parlor, and a number of classrooms. We chose to heat the whole building with electricity, and thus did not need a boiler room.

While the buildings were being constructed, the chairman of the building committee, Earle B. Roswell, acted as our overseer. Every day he and I would pore over the blueprints. One day we were looking at the side of the building facing the street and I noticed that we had a blank exterior wall. "We should impose a cross on that side," I suggested. Earle said nothing. He just took his pen and inked that cross in. The architect saw that it was added.

After we moved our church classrooms out of the farmhouse and our chapel out of the greenhouse, the chapel was left empty and the farmhouse was converted into a larger dwelling place for future use. My own family, however, had grown small: All three daughters had left and gotten married while I was still in Marshfield, and their mother, who had come up from the Vineyard to live in the parsonage for a short while, was now living in an apartment downtown and working in a bank. Finally we were quietly divorced, but we have remained friends across the years.

• • •

The Barn

Those were the 1960s: the days of youth protests and the beginnings of a new kind of drug scene. I knew a great many of the Marshfield high-schoolers from my teaching assignments and I could see their growing unrest and distrust of authority. They were experimenting with marijuana. They were protesting issues publicly. And their new ways of dressing and acting seemed so outrageous to the older generation that the gap between generations was approaching a point where it might not be reparable.

I watched as the Marshfield churches decided to do something about the situation. Coffeehouses—which featured folksingers and nonalcoholic refreshments—were popular then. Two of the churches set up coffeehouses in their church buildings and announced the hours they would be open. They provided programs to entertain the kids and chaperones to be with them.

The kids went a few times, trashed one of them, and then stopped going altogether. They were tired of authority; they hated regimentation. They felt closed in and suffocated. They wanted freedom. They protested both the rules and the adult supervision. They longed to fly. But they could not articulate their unrest.

I decided to try to help them. Some of our men renovated a large, well-constructed barn that stood behind the church's farmhouse. We put in a new tile floor and a furnace. Then we set up small tables and put candles on them . . . and it was ready for occupancy.

The parish approved, but watched developments with some apprehension as we put up a sign above the new front door—THE BARN—and waited.

Many of the high-schoolers walked by that way on their way home from school. They saw the sign and began questioning me about it. "What is it?"

"A barn," I always answered.

"What's it for?"

"It's for you. Come and look at it."

They began coming by.

After a few were gathered I would go out and tell them it was a gathering place for them, a hangout. Now they wanted to know what the program would be like. Who would oversee them? It took a while for them to become convinced that the Barn was truly for them, and that whatever activities they'd have would be the result of their initiative. That there would be no adult chaperones. That there would be no rules except those of their own making.

As the word spread, the number of attenders increased until we had more than a hundred there each night. They would knock at my door and invite me out to talk with them. They put up a tiny stage with a tall stool and a warm spotlight, and began inviting folksingers to come and entertain. Sometimes I would read poetry. While this entertainment took place they all sat on the floor quietly, except for the times they were applauding.

They brought me a list of their self-imposed rules. There would be no smoking in the barn, no drugs were to be used, no alcohol, and no "funny stuff." I am convinced that they never broke any of these rules.

The town objected to the Barn. This was not the way to run a coffeehouse, they said. Where were the adult chaperones? What were those kids doing? What kind of a man was this Methodist minister? But the people of my church never openly criticized me for this project.

One Sunday the kids asked to attend church. I think they were trying to show their appreciation. They sat together in the balcony and were all set to retreat down the hill to their Barn after the service when my people ushered them all into Ellis Hall and gave them a light lunch.

The Barn was an active drop-in center for about eighteen months. The kids would envision parties and dances but these activities never took place. They had neither the skills nor the organization nor the acceptance of individual responsibility to make the events happen. If I was sitting with them when they talked about having a party I would never butt in and steer them to use the usual committee structure that was the method of the society they protested against.

Once, the teens walked down the middle of the street to a small park. Traffic was routed around them. I walked behind them and watched. When they arrived at the park, they simply broke up and went home.

Their unrest was largely ignored. As time went on, fewer and fewer came to their drop-in center. They had found that authority and rules and structure and responsibilities were an indelible part of our social system and they would have to comply or be lost. They learned the power of "the norm."

Those kids who frequented the Barn were loyal to me. They knew I had gone out on a limb to allow them to operate this drop-in center without adult supervision. They put my picture in their high school yearbook and called me Pop Bieber. They liked to hear stories about my adventures in the military service and concluded that I was a maverick, but a maverick who operated boldly for the sake of a cause. They saw how I had stepped outside the norm, and this was the way they said they wanted to live, too. They encouraged me to continue to follow the beat of my own drummer, and supported my efforts to help during those troubled times, when their generation and mine rarely spoke civilly to each other.

For the kids in Marshfield in 1969, I was able to write letters of recommendation to help them get into college, stay in touch throughout the years, and even, eventually, officiate at their weddings when they became ready to take spouses. In retrospect I am sure that, though I never spoke to those kids about my desire to become a spiritual healer, they would have championed this dream as well.

The very real bonding between us was, I think, the basis for a person-to-person style of ministry that would later blossom in my assignment to Spencer, Massachusetts, and become part of the process of my being gifted to heal others. My response to the need of those teens, and my involvement with them through the Barn, added immeasurably to my commitment to people.

Walking Alone?

With my wife gone and my daughters also, my big parsonage was empty. But not for long.

One of our families had bought a large house for fifty dollars, with the provision that it be moved. A contractor was found who gave them a price to move it and they had a lot ready. But in order to do this they had to saw the house in half and move it in two sections. Before long the first half was moved, preceded by workers representing utilities whose wires had to be moved out of the way. The roads were closed while this was being done and half their new home was subsequently set into place. It looked odd, to say the least. But that's where the project stopped.

The contractor took weeks to arrange to bring the second half. In the meantime the family had no place to go. I brought them into my upstairs, where they stayed for about three months. There were five of them.

• • •

Before this family moved out, a fire broke out in one of Marshfield's rented beach cottages. The renter, a young mother of two children, was visiting neighbors across the street. She saw the flames and tried to get back into the cottage to save her youngsters. It was too late, they were burned to death.

I found this mother in the hospital with burned hands and face. Her boyfriend couldn't help; he was on duty at a nearby naval flying station. I arranged for the funeral and burial of the two children, and the couple moved in with me, occupying one of the downstairs bedrooms for several months until he was transferred and they moved away.

• • •

Jackie, one of the leading socialites of the town, president of the community Women's Club, and an officer in her church, came home one day to find her nine-year-old son and her husband gone, and a note explaining that he planned to divorce her and marry an existing girlfriend. He had gone to California, and taken their son.

Jackie went berserk, running naked into the street, wailing. She was later found in a policeman's home, where she was taking a shower after having broken in. She was committed to a mental hospital for a few weeks, and then brought back to court to face charges.

I didn't know her but someone told me about this and I attended court that day. The judge mused aloud that he simply did not know what to do with this case. Jackie stood there mute and helpless. I walked up to the bench and told the judge who I was, what my qualifications were, and that, if he dropped all charges, I would take her to my house and be responsible for her. He put Jackie in my charge and she moved in, adding to the "family" already sharing my home.

Jackie occupied another of the downstairs bedrooms and she seemed to be gradually recovering, but ever so slowly. In her mind I became her savior and she was demonstrative in her adulation.

About this time I was hospitalized with a heart attack, a myocardial infarction, and this was followed by several more trips to the hospital for heart spells. I didn't realize how deeply my health was affecting Jackie.

One evening one of the women of my church phoned Jackie while I was out. Later we could hear her pacing the floor of her bedroom. The next morning, while having coffee, two of us heard a gunshot from Jackie's room. We rushed there and found Jackie on the floor; she had obviously shot herself.

I held her, and someone called for help. The police arrived, and we took her to the hospital. Jackie soon died, however.

The woman who had phoned Jackie later told me what she had said. She had told Jackie that my heart problems were the result of tension . . . and that she (Jackie) was the major cause of the tension. It was sadly apparent that Jackie had decided to remove this cause, and that the caller seemed oblivious to her own need for remorse.

• • •

We set up a bedroom in the basement and an elderly recluse, a lifelong bachelor and alcoholic, moved in. I set him up in the furniture repair business and he did very well during the times when he was sober. He stayed with me for two years.

• • •

I spent seven years in Marshfield, building a church, making countless calls to invite new members, and working with teens and others in need. The Barn eventually outlived its usefulness except as a place where the homeless could occasionally come and make a stopover, which they did, never creating any problem or doing the property any damage. At the end of those seven years I was physically weaker, and I took the advice of friends that it was time to leave Marshfield. The church was making regular payments on its mortgage, and it was ready for a more conventional, less controversial pastor. So I applied to the conference for a new appointment.

The work with the Barn's teens had called for an intimate awareness of persons and their needs, despite external appearances or societal divisions. Bringing people into my home to live with me had involved both the risk of taking on personal responsibility for them and an understanding of their suffering. All this, I would later see, was part of God's plan to hone me for labor with persons on a much deeper level than many bring to either the ministry or to the practice of psychology. The gift of spiritual healing, when it came, would immerse me so deeply in a dedication to others that service to others would become my very reason to exist.

GLASTONBURY (1974–1982)

The next appointment offered me was Hazardville, Connecticut. This was meant as a reward for the work done in Marshfield, for Hazardville was one of the larger churches in the conference. It was operating smoothly, had a wonderful parsonage, a great staff, and prestige in the community. The Hazardville church had stated that they thought it would be nice to have a preacher like me, with a reputation as a good soloist and maybe even an evangelical. Consistent with my vow to serve only churches that paid the conference minimum, however, I prevailed upon the district superintendent to send me to Glastonbury instead.

Here there were two churches within five miles of each other with no pressing problems to be solved. One was an old church with families who had been going there for years and who were used to being where they were. This church was in rural East Glastonbury, outside Glastonbury Center, which was rapidly growing but not in that direction. The other church, Asbury, was a new downtown church that served Pratt-Whitney Aircraft's engineers and the insurance company workers from across the river in Hartford. Asbury was a small A-frame church with an average attendance of fifty; it had no financial problems, and the whole congregation fit into one mold of "people who belonged."

Soon after I got there, though, calamity struck. The aircraft company summarily transferred hordes of its engineers to Florida in a matter of weeks. Asbury lost its whole choir, its organist, its teachers, and 80 percent of its membership. The remaining church members felt defeated.

I set out to unite the two churches by selling Asbury and persuading its members to worship at East Glastonbury's older church. This was accomplished but with the loss of several families who chose to go to another downtown church rather than to rural East Glastonbury.

We were fortunate to sell the Asbury church to an independent group, and the parsonage through a real estate firm. We paid off the mortgages and repaid the Board of Missions of the United Methodist Church for the funds they had provided for the establishment of Asbury. Because of the sale of Asbury property and because so many Asbury families transferred to East Glastonbury, we found ourselves with a substantial sum of money to revitalize the three-story parsonage that stood next to that church. We put siding on the church building, began the restoration of the old pipe organ, and banked a comfortable sum for future projects.

After discovering that two nursing homes in Glastonbury did not have regular church services for the patients to attend, I developed an energetic nursing-home ministry. I scheduled services weekly and acquired a team to help me. I discovered early in this ministry that I needed to focus those services and those visits on individuals as much as I could. I did so, in part, because of a story I had been told.

It seemed that a group of church ladies somewhere had decided to have a party for the patients at a local home. They led them in singing, provided some entertainment, and gave each patient a little basket of goodies. One of the church ladies was so thrilled at the reception they had received on this visit that she determined to visit the home again. And so she did, a couple of weeks later. She brought a tape to play and some goodies to distribute. She found the patients in their usual seats in the large living room—each in his or her own place. A few were watching television but most just sat there while the hours passed by, their heads sunken forward and no one talking to anyone.

The churchwoman walked into the center of the room. One little lady struggled to her feet, approached her, and asked, "Did you come to see *me*?" The visitor was taken aback at this approach and she murmured, "Well, I came to see all of you." The little old lady burst into tears and shuffled slowly out of the room.

I was sure that the individual approach was what God wanted me to use, and I experimented and watched the results. When I visited nursing home groups, I would often sing with them (since I love to sing). As we sang, I would go to each patient and speak to him or her by name, aware of how easy it is to lose your identity as a patient in a nursing home. I found that when I led them in singing I could go to one who was not participating, lean over, and tell that dear soul that I wanted to hear him or her sing. Over and over the nursing-home residents responded—even, much to the surprise of the attendants, those who had never been heard to join such activities.

I drew my inspiration from the ministry of Jesus, which was largely spent with individual persons. His greatest sermon, the Sermon on the Mount (Matthew 5), was preached to

His disciples. He did not bring healing through groups, either, I had noticed; He healed a series of individuals. For example, He took a man who was a deaf-mute apart from the crowd before He signed to him that He was going to heal his speech and hearing. I decided then that, if and when I received the gift of spiritual healing, there would be no waving my arms about, no sprinkling holy water in an arc over some group seeking to be healed. I would use the individual touch: the laying on of hands. So, since I had not yet been given the gift to spiritually heal people, I would use this personal kind of ministry with my present flock.

The style of my hospital calls changed, too, because of this focus. I would not go to the bedside with a somber expression, read from my Bible, and offer a canned prayer. Instead I would offer encouragement by my confident demeanor and by my words to the individual who was ill, words that would be as positive and cheerful as I could make them.

I remember calling on one man, the husband of a regular churchgoer, a man who himself was not "religious." When I walked up to his bed he said defensively, "Have you come to pray for my soul and give me the last rites?" I replied, "Hell, no! I just wanted to say hello and see how you're doing." "Fine," he said in a more kindly tone, "sit down and we'll talk."

・・・

As I watched the results of ministering in this individual way to the ill and to the elderly and to others too, I saw encouraging results. The members of that newly merged East Glastonbury congregation were becoming more involved in their own spiritual growth than they were in their church's numerical growth. We brought back some fallen members and had a good parish. I stayed with them for eight years. Though I didn't know it at the time, it was a time of final preparation for me.

It is obvious to me now that, in Glastonbury, I was being steered farther along in the direction of God's infinite love (we call it *grace*) for individual persons. It would not be long before God would be able to gift me to bring miracles to a host of His "ones."

SPENCER (1982–1988)

My last assignment before I officially retired was to Spencer, Massachusetts. The Methodist church there is on Main Street in the center of the small town with two industries. Most Spencer residents commuted into Worcester, a few miles away, to work. The church is small and lovely. I spent the first summer there painting the downstairs classrooms. But before the fall season began, I visited the official membership. I enjoyed working with these people; they were very receptive to my ideas, and anxious to make their church a force in their lives and in the lives of others.

The conference had to contribute toward my salary for part of the first year. The congregation had fallen upon hard times and had to borrow money to pay the departing minister's salary. They had no money to cover my moving costs, so I rented a truck. Two parishioners, Howie Wilson and Herb MacMillan, were there at the parsonage to greet me and move me in.

I got off to a "good" start at the first administrative board meeting by usurping Herb's job as chairman and announcing that we would hear no reports of our financial position. That had always been the discouraging start to their meetings. Ray Harsha, church treasurer, was appalled. He had always provided detailed copies of the church's income and outgo, highlighted by what he called the "shortfall."

The rest of the finance committee was completely chagrined when I suggested that we should not go out for financial pledges in order to set the budget that year. Where would the money come from? committee members asked. How could we make a budget without knowing what people were going to give? A desperate letter of protest of my high-handed methods was fired off to our DS (district superintendent). The DS did not reply to their letter, and later told me he had been confident I had something worthwhile in mind.

Without pledges, we made up a budget of what it was going to cost us to operate the church for a year, made copies of it, and mailed the copies to our member families along with a smaller envelope. These envelopes contained a pledge card marked, *Our Pledge to God.* The envelopes were already addressed to the church and a stamp was attached.

When the pledges arrived back at the church, I announced that they would remain unopened. The people were pledging to God's work, I suggested, and none of our finance people or anyone else needed to know what the amount was.

After three or four months our finance secretary added up our income from the offering envelopes that came in each Sunday. The giving of the membership had increased 34 percent! And the budget we had made in faith was oversubscribed. The still-unopened envelopes were given back to the pledgers.

This method of meeting our budget needs was not a standard practical method. It wasn't found listed in the methods of stewardship suggested for fund-raising. Its success depended upon faith alone. So, in a way, does the success of a healing ministry, which requires a Peter willing to leap out of the boat and walk on water.

Early in my time there, the Spencer church group grew rapidly into a caring family. It was a source of joy to come to church or to attend one of our fellowship functions. Attendance at service grew and remained steady. One of the most popular services was held on Christmas Eve.

On Christmas Eve I invited families to come to the sanctuary between five and seven o'clock. Each family was brought forward to the altar, where I awaited them and knelt with them as they communed as a family group. By seven-thirty the church would be filled for our candlelight service. It featured worshipers bringing their individual candles to be lit from the large Christ cross, and when all the candles were lit and lights turned off, we sang "Silent Night" together. (I need to mention that one of our trustees was on the local volunteer fire department, and he always sat in the back with a fire extinguisher.)

• • •

Like many churches, the Spencer church was always having special projects and we needed volunteers to carry them out. Since they were of a varied nature, no one committee could be relied upon to assume responsibility for them all. So I tried another method, one which I explained after puzzling our DS one day when she stopped by on her way to a meeting.

I was sitting in my office and she passed by our bulletin board on her way in. She came in, greeted me, and then backed out, facing the board. She took down a poster and brought it to me. "What is this?" she asked.

"What does it say?" I responded.

"It says 'Sign-up Sheet' and there are forty-eight names on it."

"Yes, that's right," was all I offered.

"But what are they signing up to do?" she persisted.

"They don't know yet. We haven't decided what we're going to do," I said, proud of our members' willingness to help out, no matter what.

• • •

Sometimes the church raised money for various causes. The youth group wanted to make a small trip, and their funds were low. I decided to help them. So I bought four cases of canned peas and placed them on the altar steps. Everyone saw them there but no one ventured to ask what they were for.

During our service, after the other announcements, I gave a mock impassioned plea. It went something like this: The pea crop in Georgia had failed. The stores had sold out of their stock. No more peas were available. I had sensed that something like this was going to happen, so having foresight of my people's future needs, I had stocked up for my friends. . . . After the service the peas sold out at one dollar per can, and the kids got their money. Yes, it's true: Everyone realized it was a scam, but my attempt at levity loosened the purse strings.

• • •

I coined a word at Spencer: *fervisis*. It became popular with the folks. We were having such fun administering the affairs of the church (a task which I had always found boring) that we changed our administration to streamline it. Anyone could attend any committee meeting he or she chose. All progress worked this way: Someone would come up with an idea he or she needed help in developing. We would announce a meeting of the Fervisis Committee. Anyone at all was free to attend and enter the discussion. After this particular idea was put into action, the Fervisis Committee ceased to meet until another need arose.

A Fervisis Committee planned and brought about a week of evangelistic services. Another inaugurated a number of adult Adventure Groups. Still another planned and held a fall fair, at which there were many workers.

• • •

For one charity we wanted to support, we discarded the idea of taking a special offering. I went to a druggist and begged a lot of small pill bottles. A lady filled them with water from the church kitchen sink. We then labeled the bottles FERVISIS WATER. These were offered for sale at one dollar a bottle. We made certain that people knew what they were buying. The water had no healing value or magic potion. It wasn't good for anything, but it cost a dollar because we had the only ones available. We sold several hundred of these and some came back to be refilled. Some were sent as gifts to friends and relatives. Strangers who attended a spaghetti supper saw them, asked about them, and bought two or three bottles, grinning all the while. Some are still in existence.

• • •

For another project Carl Harling and I put on a public spaghetti supper and sold tickets. We asked people who had never worked on a church supper to volunteer. They did. Carl and I went to grocery stores and bought jars of spaghetti sauce of all kinds. We added some Italian sausage and that was it. We had a lot of inquiries about our recipe, which, we assured them, was not available. Prominent on the hall wall was a sign:

Please do not bring attention to any foreign material you may find in your food. We may not have enough of this to go around.

• • •

In Spencer I augmented my income by commercializing my hobby of refinishing furniture and caning chairs. I could do this early in the morning because I was usually up by 3 A.M. The owner of Salem Cross Inn asked me to do some work on some chairs with canvas backs that they used around tables in the summertime. He told me that the rain always ruined the finish. He brought three for me to try refinishing and then came back and got them. I had scraped off the finish, put on a light stain, and then applied several coats of paste wax that I'd buffed. No rain would bother that finish. He was delighted when he picked them up, and asked if I would do several more. A week later a truck brought seventy-five! I also did a lot of work for my friend Dave Ekleberry at the Spencer Country Inn.

Thus, with a little creativity, I was able to help provide funds to help persons in need. Today I make no charge for healing at any time. No offerings are taken. When inquiries are made, I say, "I didn't heal you. God did: Pay Him."

PART III

Whom God Empowers

Responding to the Call

In the mainline Protestant denominations, ordination comes to candidates after careful preparation and the approval of boards and committees whose responsibility it is to see that the ordinand is a proper candidate and is truly called to be a minister. At the end of this process, ordination takes place. It is characterized by the laying on of hands by elders who have that responsibility. This ritual symbolizes the church's recognition that the individual is now set aside for the work of the ministry of the church.

There exists no such formal process for recognizing those who have those special God-given gifts listed in Ephesians. In particular, the spiritual gift of healing is formally recognized by churches only reluctantly, after a preponderance of evidence shows that God's power is, indeed, present in the touch of the healer. Even then, this recognition does not often come from denominational heads. This is partly because most churches have no program of gifted healing in effect. With no such program outlined, they also have no criteria for recognition of healers. This is a sad state of affairs! Recognition of the gift of spiritual healing, then, most often comes informally, from those who have been healed.

Paul's letter to the Ephesians (3:7–9; 4:11–13) speaks of the calling to a specific ministry as a gift of God's grace. In the biblical record we see God choose many persons—kings, champions, prophets—to perform selective functions for Him. Jesus, for example, called twelve to be his closest disciples. God still calls us. And He still gives specific gifts when He calls, as He did in Paul's day.

Paul speaks of these specific gifts in I Corinthians 12:4–11. In verse 7 he says, "The Holy Spirit displays God's power through each of us as a means of helping the entire church." Then he lists some of the special gifts. In verse 9 he says, "He gives special faith to another, *and to someone else the power to heal the sick*" [emphasis added].

It should be noted that these special gifts were not meant to be confined to Old Testament times or to the early church. Nor are they meant today to be confined to clergy or to men only.

My role as a counselor or therapist was not the result of an infant form of the gift of healing that God gave me later in life. Counseling has its place; I still counsel people today. But spiritual healing is separate from it.

The difference between spiritual healing and counseling is very clear. The goal of counseling is to work out an analysis of the problem, try to deal with the causes of the dysfunction, and improve the individual's sense of well-being. A kind of success does sometimes result in the dysfunctional person's becoming integrated and confident. But this level of improvement results from the skill of the counselor and the active participation of the "client." Counseling is a process that both counselor and client can work at and improve. In counseling, the effort of the participants, the training of the counselor, matter.

In spiritual healing brought about though a gifted one, God is the One Who acts. He uses one person to bring His loving grace to another person, the receptor. The methods of bringing God's healing to the sick person are prayer (petition), and the laying on of hands. When God is asked to heal, He sometimes does and sometimes does not heal. The sick person presents him- or herself to God as desirous of healing; the healer petitions God and passes on the healing when God grants it. Effort and training do not affect the process of spiritual healing. Openness often does. And thus the presence of a person gifted as a spiritual healer helps.

I have always firmly believed in the calling by God and in the gifting by God. As I said at the outset, I prayed for more than forty years that God would give me the gift of healing. It came unexpectedly but unmistakably.

In January 1985 I was reading the letter of James again and came upon a passage I had read many times before (James 5:13–15). This time, however, it held special meaning to me.

"Is any among you suffering? He should keep on praying about it. Those who have reason to be thankful ought to be singing praises to the Lord. Is anyone sick? He should call for the elders of the church and they should pray for him and pour a little oil upon him, calling on the Lord to heal him. And their prayer, if offered in faith, will heal him, for the Lord will make him well; and if his sickness was caused by some sin, the Lord will forgive him."

I felt strangely moved after this reading. This was certainly my summons. I suddenly knew, as strongly as I could know at the time, that God was answering my prayer of almost forty years. And that my life was about to change dramatically because I would respond to that gift.

The inevitable question we humans ask about such wonders is, Why? Why me, and why at that time?

I know the answer will always be partly mysterious—we are not meant to fully understand the will of God. But I also think the answer in my case has something to do with my willingness to do what God inspired me to do. As I traveled through one stage of serving Him to another, I developed the courage to do what had to be done without waiting for someone to give me approval or resources. I learned to depend on God and accept the consequences, whether they were good or bad in the eyes of us mortals, whether they brought *me* praise or ridicule from people around me or from the church. I was becoming more and more God-centered. To use a cliché, I was willing to be a fool for Christ.

In addition, I had learned that ministry was most effective when practiced one on one. I guess I would sum it up this way: I responded to the Spirit's inspiration most of the time. Over the years, that continuing response led me to grow into a person who could receive the particular spiritual gift I craved.

I do not think that my being a minister was essential to my receiving the gift. Nor should my gift be as unusual as it is.

Many churches, particularly the Protestant Episcopal Church, have historically included in their programs services for healing and the laying on of hands by groups of people.

The Order of Saint Luke, an organization of clergy devoted to a program of healing, has fostered this form of group healing for many years and it has been successful. The Order has been reluctant, though, to recognize specific persons as having been given the distinct gift of healing. It teaches the efficacy of a person's receiving miracles through group prayer and through the touch of practitioners. As far as I know, no one member of this group has ever claimed to possess the spiritual gift of healing, however.

It is a fact that authentic healing does take place through other mediums, such as Indian shamans, gurus, masters of the Japanese method of Reiki (a Japanese system of healing by moving hands around the body), and so forth.

The inescapable, thrilling reality is that God *desires* people to be well. When they are open to His offer of a cure through what may be considered a miracle, a cure almost always takes place. Because of barriers within people, however, a healer often comes in handy to help overcome whatever is blocking a person's healing and to bring God's healing to him or her.

It is my hope that mainline Protestant churches will come to see that this spiritual gift of passing on God's healing is meant to be as abundant today as it was in the early church. If our churches would put away their fear, they could find a way to formally recognize healers who are shown to have the gift. This recognition could then be withdrawn if abused. Our churches could also incorporate healing service rites that avoid hysteria. In these ways, our churches could encourage spiritual healing, which God so obviously desires.

I have already talked about the beginning of my own healing ministry. God continues to call me to heal individuals. I continue to answer despite my infirmity and despite any continuing obstacles. My wife, Monte, is at my side, equally dedicated. What a wonderful blessing she is to me and others! At our healing services the service's length is determined only by the number of persons in the healing line waiting to be healed.

Some insights about this calling to heal that I've discovered through experience follow, in the form of questions and answers.

Questions and Answers About Spiritual Healing

The whole subject of spiritual healing brings up a lot of questions. I list some of those questions here, and give the best answers I can.

Q: *Who is the healer?*
A: The person termed in this book a spiritual healer is, of course, not the healer. That person is acting as an agent of the Holy Spirit, Who heals all. I have tried to shed light on how God chooses who His healers are, by looking at my own forty-year journey in Part II of this book. I do not, though, pretend to say that another person's journey to the gift of spiritual healing—or that the strengths and weaknesses of other such gifted people—will be the same as mine. I offer my journey as food for thought.

Q: *What are the prerequisites for spiritual healing to occur?*
A: As stated earlier in this book, God sometimes says no to requests for healing, but in my experience people are

healed about 80 percent of the time. Some of those who are not healed are not healed because of blocks they themselves put in the way of healing. And some of those blocks are a result of failures of the churches that have, at times, put more emphasis on our guilt than on the fact that we are children of God, loved beyond understanding.

The prerequisites for spiritual healing to occur are simple. Healing is not something earned because the ill person has "enough" faith, or is good enough, or prays enough, with or without friends, to merit God's attention and favor.

Healing is clearly a gift of God, a demonstration of God's love for us—a love so vast, so undeserved, that we can use only one word to describe it: *grace.* A proper understanding of God's role in the process of healing is needed.

In our world, which is so materialistic, so devoid of the personal affirmation of the nature of brotherly love, we often find ourselves thinking that God's love falls far short of our individual need. *So God is love,* we may say, *what is that to me? That kind of love is not enough for me; it's unsatisfying, too distant.* The reason we tend to think like that is simply this: We don't understand how personal God's love is. Remember the story of Jesus noticing Zacchaeus up in a tree, trying to see the Lord as He walked down the road? The story tells us, not that Zacchaeus called out to Jesus, but that *Jesus summoned Zacchaeus* down from the tree. Jesus walked into Zacchaeus's house for dinner, an uninvited guest, and then into Zacchaeus's life. Not the other way around. That passage ends with the words "I, the Son of Man, have come *to seek* and save those like him who are lost" (Luke 19:9 NLV).

On another occasion Jesus said, "Behold, I stand at the door and knock: If anyone hears and answers, I will come in and dwell with him" (Revelations 3:20).

The biggest obstacle to healing in "good" Christians is simply their inability to stop trying so hard to be faithful, to stop feeling guilty. They find it difficult to begin to say with confidence that they want to be healed, to feel God's overwhelming love *for them,* and to simply be open to it. I believe that our churches are largely responsible for this inability because of their emphasis on sin and guilt and because of their nitpicking over theology.

One dear man I remember particularly would eagerly approach me at his turn in the healing line at our healing services. He would tell me he had spent the week working on his faith so that tonight his request would be honored. It was not. This man lived alone; he was a recluse. He had no friends and no family. He had never been led to the self-fulfilling thought that God loved him and would heal him *without any price paid.* It is as though God looks askance at the one who approaches him with a basketful of faith as a price for admission to health. God requires only a trusting attitude: "A little child shall lead them" (Isaiah 11:6).

I would like to see our churches change their emphasis to one that helps people experience God's love.

Q: *Does the Christian church have a monopoly on divine healing?*
A: No, it doesn't. God heals, but there are names for God other than the ones Christians use. Christians believe in Jesus as God's Son and the Way to God. Some other world religions, and some healing programs in vogue of late, are taking the long way to get there, but their efforts are not ignored by God.

What a *shock* it can be to discover that we don't possess exclusive rights to eternity—or to healing. God is beyond the petty arguments that separate us religiously. He does not limit His love—or healing—to those who are of a chosen few.

Q: *Can a person heal him- or herself?*
A: Assuredly yes. There's a joke among ministers that we are in one of the few professions working to make ourselves unnecessary. If everyone were good, we priests or parsons

would not be needed. Similarly, a spiritual healer would not be needed if the ill individual could overcome his or her obstacles and come to God for healing with the trust of a child.

Healers *are* unnecessary for those who have found their own uncluttered avenue to God. The first step to that path was referred to by Francis Thompson. In his poem "The Hound of Heaven," we learn that God is the seeker and we are the ones sought after. The person in the middle of a great personal crisis needs only to admit exhaustion and cry out before he or she will hear the whisper in his or her ear, saying, "I'm here and I hear. Be still and know that I am God." (Read Psalm 46:10.)

God does not withhold His miracles of healing because of which religious faith a person claims (or doesn't claim). Nor does He even require a healer as an intermediary. God is waiting for us to let Him be the God of Love to us.

Q: *If a person can heal him- or herself, how does that person go about it?*
A: The prerequisites are simple yet difficult to accept because they are simple. To repeat: Accept these facts as truth: God loves you as an individual and is concerned about all your illnesses and woes. Moreover He is *anxious* to heal you.

You don't have to assail His ears with passionate and prolonged praying. You don't have to justify yourself as a candidate. You certainly don't have to bargain. You don't have to aspire to sainthood. There's *nothing* you can do to earn His miracles anyway, so, as the current saying goes: "Get a life." That is, ask Him to get you a new life with that ailment gone, that personal relationship restored, that confidence and joy in living reborn. Keep your request to God simple and confident. Then live your confidence in God's love as fully as possible. This confidence will lead you to be proactive with doctors.

If you have a chronic illness, if you face an operation to remove all or part of one or more of your organs, make sure *you* are part of the process. Ask many questions. What can you expect of this surgery? What are the side effects of the operation, the hidden risks? What are the dangers in taking these drugs? Get a second opinion. Then go step by step through the entire process as one directly and willfully involved. Be a partner with the medical authorities. Self-healing can partly depend on your participation with medical authorities on the course of action decided upon.

Recent reports of the treatment of AIDS include stories of some who have delayed the advance of this dread disease by their own mental attitude toward it. They willfully assume a positive way of living, living as though they did not have this condition. They maintain a healthy outlook and talk about their affliction as little as possible. Some have lived many months without evidence of progress of the disease. It has *not* become their identity; they have not surrendered. Why does this attitude make a difference? How is it related to spiritual self-healing?

Wholeness comes from wanting it; healing from the desire to be healed. Progress comes from wishing it were so, assuming the right attitude, being receptive. This attitude affects more than we understand, and God works with it.

Sometimes our closest friends and relatives can be unintentional blocks to our recovery from an illness. Their comments and their demeanor suggest that we should not expect miracles to happen to us. I have been in the room of a person who, comatose, heard a visitor —a member of the family—discuss the appearance of the patient in despairing tones, thus casting an air of gloom in the sickroom. Since comatose people—though unable to communicate— can often hear what is said, the sick person exposed to such comments must overcome the insidious disparagements from these prophets of doom. It is difficult to be positive and believe in miracles if no one close to us believes. But in order to heal yourself, you need to continue to believe that, yes, you *can* be healed.

This positive approach is essential in self-healing; we must be able to offset the negative influences of others. I remember taking a walk through the woods with my brother when I was small. We came to a stream we thought we should cross to see what was on the other side. We didn't want to wade and there were no stones to step on. Charles assured me we could jump it, and I believed him. He went up a hill and then came flying down, jumped, and landed safely on the other side. He told me to come on over. I went up the hill, came running down, and—just as I was about to make the great leap—he shouted, "You won't make it!" I didn't. I was not able to put aside his negative attitude quickly enough.

I remember two brothers, both in their seventies, both with cancer of the bowels, both in the hospital at the same time. One was an elder in his church and had frequent visits from his family. The other lived alone and supposedly had no religion. The church-connected brother died, unable to believe he was going to be healed. The other brother lived. He never doubted that he would win out over this dread disease. He healed himself through his positive attitude, through his desire for health—and by God's grace, which he did not acknowledge.

Think of your own healing process this way: If you pray many times a day to get well, you are acknowledging the presence of your problem every time you name it, bringing it to your own attention. This habit can have a negative effect on your program of self-healing. While you cannot be expected to forget your pain and your concern, you only reinforce your problem when you overdo your praying. God is not deaf, nor does He get pleasure from our pleading.

Be proactive in what you can do physically to improve the problem. Place the problem in God's hands, believe that you are important to God. Then trust that He will heal you, no matter what anyone else says. If you cannot get past whatever obstacles there are between you and God's healing, that is the time to ask a spiritual healer to bring God's healing to you.

Q: *Can I hope to become a spiritual healer?*
A: Yes, it is possible. God still calls persons to do His bidding, and the need for healers is widespread. As I mentioned earlier, a number of qualities are needed in a healer.

The first is courage. In an Old Testament story, God called one man for a heroic assignment but the man demurred. Gideon said he was a member of the lowest tribe in Israel and he was the lowest in his tribe! Why would God choose him? One needs to be convinced that the call of God is real and personal and insistent. Gideon did cooperate with

God. Moses led the people of Israel out of Egypt. It takes courage to believe that you can heal in God's name.

Next, to be a healer one needs to be an obedient servant. *The healer* does not heal; healing occurs through the power of God. It is good to ask yourself: Do you have the courage to believe that you can work miracles for God? Will you step forward to offer healing without hesitation and with a strong faith that success will follow? Can you announce yourself publicly as a vessel, a conduit through whom God works?

Peter had that courage when he jumped out of the boat to be with Jesus when he saw the Lord walking across the sea toward the disciples. Peter sank, but he *did* jump out of the boat. He would have been successful in walking on the water had he kept his eyes firmly fixed on the eyes of his Master.

Finally, a healer must be humble enough to remember that, when he or she sees and feels God's power working on the bodies and minds and spirits of the ones seeking healing, the healer is merely a witness to, a minor participant in, the miracles being worked. Around the time of a healing this feeling of deep humility and gratitude that God has healed is so moving that the healer tends to be overcome with thanksgiving. But later, the healer needs to remember that God uses other servants for healing too; and He uses others with other talents and gifts for other needs. Being a healer does not place the healer above other servants of God in any way.

Q: *Can a spiritual healer train someone else to be a healer?*
A: In my experience the answer is no. Spiritual healing is dependent upon the gift God gives. A healer cannot give that gift. I do think that if a person feels he or she has been given the gift to heal, a healer could help him or her with some insights from experience.

On one occasion a pastor came to me and tearfully said he wanted to become a healer. He was convinced he was ready to dare to do this. I suggested he come to the next healing service and stand near me while the line proceeded. He did. At one point I stepped over to him and asked him to lay his hands upon the seeker with me. He panicked. He burst into tears and returned to his seat in the pews.

Q: *Does a spiritual healer ever work with other healers? Why or why not?*
A: Though I have never had that opportunity, I would welcome it. Through the years of my healing ministry in New England I have known only three Roman Catholic healers

and no United Methodist healers who use the laying on of hands as I do.

Q: *How does a spiritual healer prepare him- or herself for a healing service?*

A: I do so by much prayer, by not eating any meal that day except for a minor source of nourishment. By remaining outside the sanctuary in prayer while the early part of the service is taking place. By advancing to the altar just before the healing line forms, and by presenting my hands as I face the cross and ask for a special renewal of my validity to transmit God's healing power.

Q: *How long do the effects of a healing last?*

A: There is no "expiration date" on spiritual healing. I have kept in touch with a number of people who have received healing and none of them have had a recurrence of that particular problem. Some, of course, have fallen ill with other illness, or with a related illness but not in the same area.

Q: *Can a person be healed in advance—sort of an immunization against illness or accident?*

A: A healing prayer or an anointing does not provide some magic shield that protects you from future harm. It is not an inoculation. It does acknowledge dependence on God's grace and ask for His blessing in any given situation. In the mind and spirit of the seeker, it provides an atmosphere in which frantic apprehension is no longer experienced.

Q: *Is it all right to request healing for someone who doesn't ask for it?*

A: Certainly. A person making this request is acting as an agent of God according to *his* or *her* faith in God's personal love. I sometimes pray with a person seeking help for someone not present and not involved, by asking God to perform an invasion of love within that person.

Q: *If a doctor enlists a spiritual healer's help, does the spiritual healer ask the doctor to pray with him or her?*

A: I always do. When I am in the room with a doctor and his or her patient in the hospital, I pray aloud for the patient. The doctor stands next to me and signifies to the patient that he or she *expects* the prayer to be answered.

Q: *Can the gift of spiritual healing go away if it's not used?*

A: Yes, I think so. In 1988 I foolishly retired and moved with my family to Florida. I had been in Florida only eight days when, as I was sitting by the pool one day, a youth walked by with a growth on his leg. I saw that as a reminder from

God that, though I was no longer an active minister, He still expected me to use His gift for His children in need. I stopped the boy at the pool, laid my hands on the growth, and prayed that it be healed. The growth disappeared instantly. I then called an airline for a trip back north. The gift of healing should not be put in a box and stored away. *I will always use my gift of healing.*

Q: *Does a person given such an obvious gift as spiritual healing become a perfect person?*
A: No. While a spiritual healer must remain faithful to the gift, God allows His healer to retain his own unique personality. I have never presented myself as a pious, mysterious presence. For example, I cannot keep from using humor in the healing process. A teenage girl came for a healing of a head cold. I suggested that she go out in the snow, get pneumonia, and come back for healing. She saw the grin on my face, and stood steadfast. She was healed.

What I Have Learned About Spiritual Healing

Here is a summary of what I have learned through the years:

1. Each of us is innately capable of healing ourselves in many instances. Blocks to the self-healing process are erected by an enforced skepticism created by the secular society in which we live, and by confused religious training.

2. When we cannot bring about this healing on our own, the prayers of others—most notably, the prayer and the touch of one gifted with the power to heal as God's agent—can break through the barrier and effect a cure. Such a healing is still solely the work of the Holy Spirit.

3. Though no person should be regarded as incurable or any disease outside the scope of God's power to heal, it is also true that not every person who comes for healing will be healed. Sometimes the ill person's internal barriers to healing are deeply entrenched, so the door is not opened. Other times, God simply says no. There will always be mystery in the will of God, but it should be remembered that "God is not willing

that any should perish but that all should have everlasting life" (2 Peter 6:9). And that God has also said, "Behold, I stand at the door and knock. If anyone opens the door I will come in and dwell with him" (Revelation 3:20).

It must be noted, too, that death is a healing measure. This is not the place to discuss the pros and cons of euthanasia ("mercy killing"), but it is clear that there *are* times when it is a blessing for someone elderly, helpless, or physically miserable to pass on to the heavenly realm. At such times it is easy to see that death is, indeed, a victory.

I was asked to telephone Julia, a woman in South Carolina, and pray with her for healing. It was Julia's daughter who asked me, and until she asked, I knew neither of them. Julia had been given two weeks to live. She was wracked with cancer and in palliative care. She had been operated on and had gone through courses of both chemotherapy and radiation. The first thing I did when I called was to explain that her daughter had asked me to call and pray with her. Julia was calm and appreciative, polite and warm. When I asked if I could pray with her, she readily assented but suggested that my prayer ask God for a peaceful passing. She said, "You know, death itself is healing." That is how we prayed, and she passed away a month later.

4. Some people have been given the power to pass on God's healing to others. The transfer of this curative power is

characterized in the supplicant by a feeling of warmth, a sense of vibrations, and a feeling of peace that can render the one healed temporarily insensible. Many call this feeling "spaced out." The spiritual healer feels the power going from him or her into the person healed.

5. The use of oil and anointing (as described in James 5:14) is, in my experience, most effective when the sick person is bedridden or comatose.

6. Prayers offered on behalf of someone in need of healing but not present at that time are characterized by a joining of the hands or arms of the person requesting the healing and the healer. God is asked in that joint prayer to enter at that moment into the life of the person in need.

7. Faith is a factor in the healing process, but in a different way than I would have thought earlier. The individual who has been convinced that a significant amount of faith is required before he or she can receive "favors" from God is actually subverting God's gift. God does not bargain with us, measuring His gifts in proportion to our faith. The person who agonizes in an attempt to accrue the "required amount" of faith is standing in the way of healing, by focusing on the previously described erroneous list of requirements for God's attention. Healing is a gift of the grace of God. One must believe that God is always concerned and always involved. Isaiah's "a little child shall lead them" is the appropriate scriptural

direction. Take your petition to God and trust in His desire to demonstrate His love for you. I have seen many made well who had declared themselves to be unbelievers. For them, I think, faith in God is the role of the person who sent them for healing and in the person of the spiritual healer. God is, then, glorified in the unbeliever's recovery from illness or trouble. Though they acknowledge that God has healed them, I suspect that not all thank Him.

8. I do not find it difficult to admit that there are some matters about divine healing that I do not understand. I learned long ago that I cannot question God's desire to heal, His power to do so, whom He chooses to heal in a visible way, or the methods He uses. After all, I am only the servant.

Do you know the story of Jesus' first miracle at the wedding in Cana of Galilee? It is a rich story, which tells how Jesus actually began His teaching and healing ministry (John 2:1–11). He and His disciples were attending a wedding reception. Actually the story begins with the words "And there was a wedding at Cana of Galilee and the mother of Jesus was there." It continues, "And Jesus and His disciples had also been invited to the wedding." Now, according to the best principles of journalism, who is this story about? It has always been used to tell of Jesus' miraculous power: He changed water into wine. But Mary is first upon the scene. Is this a story of a mother who wanted to send her son forth on His mission?

Mary tells her son Jesus that the wedding party has run out of wine. He gives an abrupt response: Why bother Me about this? She calls the caterer's servants forward and tells them to do what Jesus commands. That's a Mother's Day sermon and I have used it as such!

But this story has other heroic figures in addition to Mary. The waiters are told to fill jugs with water and serve it as wine. How long would you last in that job, serving water as wine? But these people had looked into the face of the Christ and they did just as He bade them. The result of their faith? The wedding guests reported it to be the best wine of the evening!

So if God tells me I am to bring healing over the telephone, I will do as He commands. I will "pour from the jugs." And I do so without hesitation. My wife and I have many who phone from as far away as California and ask for healing for various physical problems. They hold the phone across their foreheads while I pray. They call me back in two or three days and register positive results!

Some Obstacles to Healing

A LACK OF LOVE OF SELF

From personal experience, from observation, and from conclusions, I have discovered some of the obstacles to healing. The biggest obstacle is the difficulty the sick or troubled person has with the idea of the God of the universe singling him or her out for special attention. "I do not deserve it." "Others are worse off than I am." "God doesn't have time for someone like me." Statements like these, often regarded as noble, are really confessions of a lack of understanding of the personal nature of God's love. The story of the Ninety-and-Nine (Matthew 18:12ff) speaks of this issue as Jesus explains the Father's regard for each individual person. Think about it! Healing is made possible when the supplicant understands his or her individual worth in the sight of God, then claims what is his or hers through the grace of God, undeserved and unearned.

How many sermons have we heard warning us against the sins of pride and arrogance and calling for humility and self-effacement! It is true that we sometimes need to be reminded that we are only human, and not God. It is worthwhile for us to be reminded that we sin, even if our sins are not the black-and-whites, but the grays.

But there are times, too, when we need to be reminded of our value in the sight of God, in the eyes of others, and in our own self-estimation. We need sermons more often on the high regard God has for us. Stories like the Ninety-and-Nine recount the worth Jesus Christ places upon the individual person. This story might also prompt us to ask what value we place on ourselves. I'm not speaking of the weakness of the human race, or of our own society, or of the religious denomination we give our loyalty to. What is your idea of yourself?

In my counseling work I have talked to thousands of people, persons who have faced me across a desk or in their own living rooms. After more than fifty years I have mentally catalogued the types of problems they have presented. And now I can conclude what the prevailing problem is. The manifestations of the problems may be different, even bizarre, but one difficulty stands out. There are a great many people alive today who either consciously or unconsciously do not like themselves. The greatest problem is the mystery of self, manifested by a lack of self-understanding and thus of self-esteem.

I would have come to this conclusion earlier in my life if I had been interested in statistics, and I would have understood it earlier if I had known then what Jesus meant when he said, "Men can be forgiven any sin and any evil thing they say, but whoever says evil things against the Holy Spirit will not be forgiven" (Mark 3: 2–9). The Holy Spirit is God within us— that spark of divinity placed within us at our creation. The person who continually says evil things against him- or herself, or who fails to say or think good things consistently, is so warping his or her soul that . . . God cannot break through to forgive and grant newness of life. Only when we recognize our own value as a person can God help us.

I think of that most poignant sentence in the familiar story of the prodigal son (Luke 15:11–32), the one in which the narrator says, "And when he had come to himself." Only when the wayward son truly looked within and decided to start on the upward path with confidence and assurance and resolution was he able to take positive action. He *did* take positive action, but not until he had faced himself, admitted his wrong, and decided to build on what he had. He was able to decide that he'd be content to be a laborer on his father's farm because he had found the nobility within his own spirit, and that was enough.

I worked alongside a giant African American years ago, digging ditches for sewer pipes. He was so good at his trade that I couldn't keep up with him. The money I earned with that good work was for my own tuition. His money supported a family. "John," I asked him one day while we were resting, "don't you want to be anything else but a ditchdigger?" He replied with a display of self-knowledge that it has taken me a long while to achieve, "Maybe, but for now I just want to be the best ditchdigger in these parts." And he sang as he worked! I doubt if he ever spent any time on a psychiatrist's couch.

Our species has spent much of the time we have been on this earth trying to solve the mysteries of the universe. We have made great strides in science and technology but we have lagged far behind in the social sciences. We have spent comparatively little time trying to understand the world of mankind. And we have spent considerably less time trying to understand ourselves as individuals. We all know of a person who is so deeply involved in the problems of others that there is no time for his or her own troubles. This is generally true: Man's greatest mystery is still . . . himself.

What a pity, since this self-understanding is so important in what matters! No one is chosen to be an astronaut because of personality. But astronauts must be supremely confident individuals who can do more than work through the complicated routines required for space travel. Astronauts must maintain objectivity and an ability to handle emergencies.

A pitcher in a World Series game must possess more than

pitching skill and cunning and speed. He must also be confident in himself in order to do a good job.

A schoolteacher may know her subject well, but she also must possess poise and confidence in herself, for the lack of these qualities is instantly communicated to the pupil who is looking for signs of weakness and ineptness, and chaos results.

A husband who is not fully in love with himself is not able to love his wife or his children. If he does not love himself, he brings less than his best to the marriage.

This understanding of who we are—lovable, though imperfect beings—is crucial to being healable. If I do not like myself, I cannot truly love God or anyone else. The moment of conversion in the religious life has been described many ways. Usually one thinks of it as a moment of complete surrender, a confession of sins, a feeling of shame, and a need to repent and make atonement. Sometimes conversion happens that way. But the most important element in conversion—and this can happen without an overwhelming sense of sin and shame—is the moment when we become convinced that God loves us . . . and thus we must be worthy of love. This realization allows us to love back in a more complete way than we could before our new understanding. From this moment the confidence grows, so that we can truly be a soldier of Christ, a fisher of men, a member of Christ's body on earth.

Paul had a conversion experience on the way to Damascus. Afterward he would say, "I am a new creature in Christ Jesus, I am not ashamed of the Gospel of Christ." And what is the Gospel, the "good news" of Christ? It is that Jesus Christ found you worthy enough to die for. In logical sequence, then, if we are worthy of Christ's love, we are worthy of our own love.

Do you love you? There are a lot of things standing in the way of this conclusion, this affirmation that we are worthy to be loved.

Blocking the way to self-understanding and thus the achievement of personhood are the same fences that obstruct the way to understanding others: Why don't I know others better? Because I haven't really tried. Because they hide themselves from me. Because my prejudices stand in the way of being really objective. Because I do not want to know them, lest the comparison between us puts me in a bad light. In the pursuit of self-knowledge these same fences exist, except they are thicker—as though made of brick, not wood—and are all the more difficult to tear down. I do not know me for the same reasons I do not know others. (Read through those reasons again!)

If you are hungry enough, you will soon find a way to eat; if you are thirsty, you will drink. If cold, you will seek shelter. These are physical needs and difficult to ignore. But to know yourself is something you can put off until another day, since you can live somewhat comfortably with the stranger who is Yourself.

It's a scary thing, at first, to investigate this self. You are always afraid of what you may find out. It is easier to go on hiding from this self-understanding than to summon the courage needed to investigate. Society has created many diversions to keep us from such meditation. Yet we must try.

Knowing one's self and loving one's self are at the heart of Christianity, as seen in Proverbs 23:7: "As a man thinketh in his heart so is he." Jesus freed us from the bonds of law and tradition and gave us up to our own consciences (those inner voices that indicate right choices). He told us to observe the spirit more than the law. He showed us that the person is more important than the crime he has committed. He asked His disciples not to look for favor among men but to find it in the sight of God—and thus in their own eyes, for they were each a temple of God's Spirit.

In order to succeed in our pursuit of that Spirit within that is good and worthy of love, we have to overcome our prejudices. Prejudices are feelings we have against someone else, they are also feelings we have against ourselves. If we know something about another that prejudices us against that person, how much more do we know things about ourselves that make it difficult to love ourselves?

We may be tempted to look only at how many times we've failed, how many evil thoughts we've harbored. We may listen to the enemies of procrastination, rationalizing, and making excuses. Why? Because we're afraid we will be disappointed in ourselves—as though our shortcomings are what matter! All these obstacles must be overcome before we can love ourselves—in the same way that they have to be overcome before we can love someone else . . . or God.

Do you see what Jesus meant by blasphemy against the Holy Spirit? Let's rephrase that verse (Matthew 12:31) this way: "You can be forgiven for any kind of sin or evil thought, but it is impossible for you to be forgiven for blasphemy against the Holy Spirit. That is God's spirit within you . . . That is *you*. If you do not love yourself you will not consider yourself worthy of God's forgiveness and God's love . . . and God's healing. It is a hopeless situation."

Therefore, when John 15:12 says, "Brethren, you ought to love one another," it also might say, "Brethren, you ought to love *yourselves*." In the love chapter (I Corinthians 13), we read, essentially, "There is nothing that love cannot face; there is no limit to its faith, its hope, and its endurance."

Remember the story of the centurion who asked Jesus to heal his ill servant? (Matthew 8:5ff) The centurion didn't want to bother Jesus enough to ask Him to come to his house, and he understood the Lord's power. In the modern-day Mass, communicants utter an affirmation similar to the centurion's reply to Jesus' offer to come to his house. They say, "I am not worthy that You should come under my roof, but speak the word and my soul shall be healed." Before they commune they admit that they are unworthy of Christ's love (and their own love), but they then place their faith in Christ and resolve to live a confident life with new strength and new love for themselves and others.

This is the spirit of love that we should be striving for. And it must be present in us before we can be healed.

**A VIEW OF ILLNESS
AS A RESULT OF INADEQUATE PRAYER**

We should already know that it is God's will for us to be well. It is a mistake to insert the words "if it be Thy will" in our prayer for healing. It *is* God's will that we be healthy. The Scriptures have many verses that attest to this fact. The whole personal ministry of Jesus Christ impresses us with the value God places upon our welfare. To ask what God's will is in this instance suggests that we do not know God.

People who are afflicted with progressive diseases tend to pray constantly for relief from their miserable state. The other persons in the household are also praying. Petitions become the focal point of their existence together. I suggest a respite from this praying for a day or two. It is best not to repeat your prayer for a cure over and over, but to utter a simple prayer of thanksgiving instead. Since God loves us, we should assume that He is at work within us. God not only loves a cheerful giver; He loves a confident pray-er.

A VIEW OF ILLNESS AS PUNISHMENT

We need also to remember that, since the New Covenant, at least, God never inflicts disease upon us as a punishment for sin. We sometimes do this ourselves, however. God takes no pleasure in our suffering. Pain is not a payment for sin. Nor does God send suffering to put us to the test to see how good we are, how patient, or how faithful. (This is a separate issue from how we react when suffering occurs.) God does not keep score on our piety level.

A DEATH WISH

It is my thesis that a large number of us possess what I call a death wish, in order to explain why we have a strong tendency to remain where we are in life rather than venture forth as a reborn person. This death wish, in varying levels of intensity, is an obstacle to spiritual healing.

The basic symptoms of the death wish are feelings that

most of us will admit to having: We don't feel like getting out of bed today; we put off that distasteful task or hold off on a decision; we decline tasks that we could do but don't really feel confident doing; we come to the conclusion that we are a person without worth; we sink into a mood of despair and despondency; we assume the identity of one who is dysfunctional because that is the way others see us . . . and on and on. Adding up the sum of these feelings, we can see how inviting actual suicide sometimes becomes.

A primary source of what I term this death wish is something I have decided to call the identity syndrome. Since the days of Freud, psychotherapists have maintained that we are all products of our past. There is still a tug-of-war between experts as to which is the *major* influence—heredity or environment. But either way, the past has important clues that can help us solve problems we develop in later life.

Call it pigeonholing, stereotyping, statistical analysis, or whatever, this problem that I call the identity syndrome is something we're all vulnerable to. Whichever factors we choose (by recollection and imagination) as being *our own* contributions to the formation of our identity, we should not leave out these few reminders of how our identity was formed by *society:* Before we are born we are identified as female or male; immediately after birth, our weight and length are heralded abroad; then the discussion begins as to which parent we most closely resemble. This is just the beginning of a vast array of society-defined factors. The next ones are: when we had our first tooth, when we took our first step, when we uttered our first words, and so on.

When we get into school we fit ourselves into a category, according to the identification given us by others. We are students who excel scholastically, hand in excellent homework on time, get on the honor roll. Or we are jocks engaged in sports, who wear clothes marked with the name of the school. Or we are the artist who dresses in the clothes we define as nonconformist, and who writes or draws or acts or creates films. Or we are cutups, always in trouble, skipping school, creating ruckuses, defying authority. Or alas, we could be misfits who fit into none of these four, who are just there, who make no claim to being in any category, who want only to be not noticed by anyone.

Why is this identity syndrome important to understand? Because it holds important clues on how a person can become dysfunctional. All of us have some dysfunction, which can be understood a little more clearly by looking at major cases.

The beginnings of major dysfunction are found in our having been categorized, one way or another. When we have a traumatic experience that cripples our psyche and labels us as helpless, many of us seek professional help. The first step is the diagnosis: Our dysfunction is given a name or several names. Then we move into the area of therapy: We are counseled weekly by a therapist. We see a psychiatrist once a month. We are medicated. We join group therapy. We may be hospitalized.

Our family and friends now have us typed as "ill" and they usually treat us carefully and sympathetically. It doesn't take long before we accept all the attempts to pigeonhole us from the time we were born. It is to this acceptance that the inception of our mental illness can be traced: We have now assimilated a new identity, that of a crippled person. This identity is, in essence, a death wish.

Moving out of this identity entails major effort. It is easier to settle down and be the sick person we "are." I have known many of these psychologically crippled people. They have come to me during a time of fleeting hope that things can change. Perhaps they think it possible that a healer can bring about a metamorphosis; possibly there is a miracle somewhere for them. But the identity is deeply entrenched and it takes me only a few moments before I sense the despair in such a person. I can always detect when this is one of those coming for help who is not going to have that necessary rebirth. I treat them kindly because I know what a gigantic effort it took to come to me after the many years in that pigeonhole. I just pray for them and ask God to get through to them: It could be so different for them.

It is good to understand this pattern of thinking, for it affects many more of us—in large or small ways—than we tend to admit. The unfortunate persons with a major death wish have cousins in so-called normal society.

One example is the hundreds of married couples whose marriages have gone stale, who ask for a way to make their lives together come alive. The element they are missing is that courage to face the issues: They need to get to know—and love—themselves and each other, and get out of whatever behavioral ruts they have fallen into. This task often seems to be an insurmountable one because they are too accustomed to settling for less than they are meant to have. And besides, the ruts are familiar. How many marriages are doomed to dullness because husband and wife have grown used to their boring existence? It takes real determination to make changes. But as with other obstacles to healing, a constant effort to be reborn is always rewarded.

Another example can be seen in John's fifth chapter, which begins with the story of how Jesus came upon a man lying paralyzed by the pool of Bethesda. Local superstition indicated that an angel stirred the water of the pool on occasion. Anyone who entered the pool at this particular time would be healed. This man had been there for thirty-eight years. Jesus walked up to him and asked, "Do you want to be healed?" The invalid answered that he had no one to help him. Jesus said to him, "Take up your bed and walk." The man did so—and was well.

What does this story say? It seems obvious that, before Jesus came to him, the man *did not particularly want to be healed.* Thirty-eight years? Someone had to be taking care of him, so it must be that his identity as a paralyzed man had become a comfortable shield. We might say of someone like him today, "He has it made." He was like those people who talk constantly about their illness, whose illness is now their identity; they are not anxious to change. We have all met this kind of person.

A young woman sat in my office one day and announced, "I am a manic-depressive and a schizophrenic." Off guard, I murmured, "Do tell." I asked her how long she had been sick. "Eighteen years." "And what has been done about it?" She described the standard therapy process of medication and counseling sessions she had been through. "And what have you come to see me for?" This appropriate question startled her. I think she suddenly realized that she had come for healing and that this man she had come to see was a healer of note. The prospect of taking on the identity of a healthy person was apparently too much for her to contemplate, for, though we talked a little while longer, she left in some embarrassment—unhealed.

Is there a solution to this most unfortunate (and widespread) situation? I believe there is: What I was yesterday I do not need to be today. There is a need for a new birthday. Do you want to be well? Then, no matter what identity people have forced upon you, no matter what happened long ago that triggered your present inability to function, no matter how seriously it has begun to hold you in a vice grip, you must decide this:

I must be well. My will is to be well. I can change. I don't have to live this way—there is happiness available to me.

Though you feel that there's no one who really cares, there is One. That one is God! He cares! He has time for you, though you feel you have not earned His love and care. You think you have not earned it? You don't deserve it? You have not "paid your dues"? You are right! *No one* can earn it—God's love is His gift to us, at no cost to us. The price, the dues, have been paid in full by His Son.

To be healed, one can follow these steps: Desire to change. Desire to be happy. Desire to be productive and giving. Accept the fact that millions attest to:

God cares for me; I will let Him help me and heal me.

And simply ask. This simple formula sums it up:

God loves me. Therefore I am lovable. Now I can love others.

That's too simple? That's the problem with real truth: It *is* simple. It's not difficult to understand why the formula that begins with the realization that God loves you *personally* is received with skepticism. The reason is the unfinished view of God that too many religionists have made part of our spiritual training. They say only that *God* is love. They do not emphasize the other part: that God loves *me.* I beg you to ask, Does God expect me to break out of this trap of victim identity that is now an old friend, and believe that I am *lovable*? My answer is, Yes. That is precisely what God wants.

Our experiences in life have taught us the opposite: We have become skeptics. We think that if we want something bad enough, we have to work hard to get it—even in the realm of God's miracles. How many times have we been foiled, cheated by schemes and projects and purchases and promises? We think we need to be wary of any person who comes along and tries to persuade us that the God of all the universe is concerned about one soul—ours. So we respond to God's offer of healing by essentially saying, *"You expect me to believe that?"*

A woman brought her teenage daughter to see me. She had about given up on the girl. She wouldn't go to school. She was into drugs. She wore a modified Mohawk haircut. She wore boots and jeans and a ragged sweater. She was overweight. I asked her mother to leave the room.

For a short while the girl and I sat and stared at each other. She had not come of her own volition and was defiant in her attitude. Finally I said, "You are a beautiful person." More silence. Then, "Why are you hiding it? Where are you going from here?" She remained silent but I could see that she was curious. She was not ready to talk, thinking perhaps, "Where is this man coming from?" I said, "I love you because you are one of God's children and He loves you. I can see that—beneath the exterior you have been careful to assume in order to fit the image people have of you—you are a beautiful girl."

Again I waited and looked away. When I looked back the tears were streaming down her cheeks. God had gotten through to her as I knew He would; I had been praying silently for her healing without the laying on of hands. The metamorphosis was complete in those few minutes. That's the way God works. I hadn't done anything. Not even the laying on of hands. This was the work of the Spirit! *A miracle!*

I brought her mother back. She saw that her daughter had been weeping. "When is the next appointment?" she asked. "She doesn't need an appointment," I said, "but she will get back to me." They left.

This newly born young lady let her hair grow back, gave up her drugs, went back to school, and graduated. I saw her a few years later in her prom gown. She has found out that God does love her, that she *is* lovable, and she has learned to share herself with others. She has kept in touch with me. I have a dozen notes from her mother expressing thanks.

A MISINTERPRETATION OF PHANTOM PAIN

Further pursuing my commitment to bring healing to those who approach me, I was not making any headway with a lady named Alice, who complained of pain in her heart. It was not relieved by the healing touch in my office. She returned several days later as I had suggested. This time I had her recount the story of her previous treatment for a heart condition. She had been seeing her doctor for several years.

I learned that she had had triple-bypass surgery several years before. After a period of recovery, the pains returned. Since then she had undergone three arterial catheterization procedures. (In this procedure an opening is made in a major artery in the groin area, a dye is injected, and a catheter is fed through the artery and into both chambers of the heart.) No more blockages were found that warranted another bypass operation, but the pain persisted. She then had three procedures of angioplasty (in which a thin tube is fed through the artery and a small balloon is inflated to clear any obstacles to the blood flow). Severe pain persisted. Her doctor was now prescribing morphine to ease the torment. What could be causing the pain?

Suddenly it occurred to me: I remembered hearing about

a phenomenon called phantom pain. This is a recognized condition that exists when someone loses a limb and the nerve endings still send a signal of pain to the brain for an appendage that does not exist. Could it be that Alice was experiencing a type of phantom pain—real, but not real?

I called her doctor and explained my theory. After some discussion of this possibility, he agreed that it might be the answer. What, then, should we do about it? We decided to attack the problem by each of us explaining what we now thought was the cause of her severe discomfort: The traumatic experience of her treatments for the problem and the recollection of pain were embedded in her subconscious mind. There was now nothing wrong with her heart or her circulatory system, but the residue of experience and memory was deeply entrenched. Each of us provided assurances that she should accept this theory.

She readily agreed to ask God to clear her subconscious mind of the phantom pain. We gave the cause to God in prayer. The morphine was withdrawn, the pain left, and she is living an active life, happy to be free. My experience in psychology provided a diagnosis; my work as a spiritual healer brought about the cure.

•••

FEARS OF CLERGY

One of the biggest obstacles to healing that I've seen is a lack of healers. This is partly due to a lack of recognition of that spiritual gift by organized churches, especially the mainline Protestant churches. I have sought to encourage churches to overcome the fear of this gift so that God can work more effectively through them.

On one occasion I was asked to address a subdistrict gathering of United Methodist clergy. My topic was titled "Spiritual Healing."

I began by announcing that I was not bringing any bibliography of reading material for them to refer to, and that I was speaking from the prejudice of personal experience in the field. I gave them some idea of my background, spoke about my commitment to the idea of healing as a special gift bestowed by God, described the gift as it came to me, and related the early experiences of my healing ministry. I quoted a number of scriptural references:

> James 5:14–16. "Is any among you sick? He should call the elders of the church to pray over him and anoint him with oil in the name of the Lord. And the prayer offered in faith will make him well, the Lord will raise him up."

> Luke 9:1–2. "When Jesus had called the twelve together, He gave them power and authority to drive out all de-

mons and to cure diseases, and He sent them out to preach the kingdom of God and to heal the sick."

Mark 9:23. "Everything is possible to him who believes." Matthew 19:26. "Jesus looked at them and said, 'With man this is impossible, but with God all things are possible.'"

I Corinthians 12:1, 4–11. "Now about spiritual gifts, brothers, I do not want you to be ignorant. There are different kinds of gifts, but the same Lord. There are different kinds of working, but the same God works all of them in all men. Now to each one the manifestations of the Spirit are given for the common good. To one there is given through the Spirit the message of wisdom, to another the message of knowledge by the same Spirit, to another faith by the same Spirit, to another gifts of healing by that one Spirit . . ."

Next I made a number of statements about theological considerations that I had found to be pertinent and vital:

- God does not test us with suffering.
- God does not punish us with illness.
- God wants us all to be well.
- There is no nobility in suffering itself.
- God does not place the burden of healing on us.

- Faith, as we have preached the need for it, plays no significant role in our "eligibility" to be cured.
- When we use the phrase "God's will be done," we are carelessly rationalizing our failure to be healed; and the fact is that God's will is that we be well.

I then launched into a discourse about what it takes for healing to occur (healing of body, mind, and spirit). I spoke of why some people are healed and others are not: Those healed, I told them, discover—some of them for the first time—how to be open to God's individual love for them. The church has long taught that God is love but has often failed to emphasize that His love is personal.

I explained that the atmosphere of one of my healing services is that of a community that has come to see God at work in the workings of miracles. As hands are laid on the petitioners, one at a time, those waiting their turn sit in the pews, praying and expectant. No attempt is made to create a mass hysteria in which the reaction is superficial and false.

Persons are healed, I said, because the power of the Holy Spirit is allowed to work within them, to bring about what God already wants and offers: wholeness and health. The role of the healer is to break down any barriers between the individual and God. As a healer, I do this through my gift and the power of my own faith in that gift.

Up to this point my presentation was well received. Perhaps I should have ended my discussion at this point. But at that time I was—and to this day I still am—disheartened at the absence of a meaningful program of spiritual healing in the yearly programs of our mainline Protestant denominations. None of my hearers at that meeting had any form of healing program in their churches. So I continued to offer the following opinion as to why ministers are not involved in obeying Jesus' command to heal.

First, I declared, many pastors are not involved in divine healing because they do not believe in it. I concurred with the Episcopal rector, whose name I have lost, who wrote, "They may be faithful in calling on the sick, fervent in prayer, and diligent in taking Holy Communion to the shut-ins. But they still do not believe that Jesus Christ heals today, through the laying on of hands and anointing with oil."

The second reason more ministers are not involved in healing, I said, is that they are afraid. One church issued me an invitation to hold a healing service and then canceled it because their board did not think this type of ministry would give the "proper image" to the community. What are clergy afraid of? I asked. And then I answered for them: They are afraid that if they become involved, they will be considered radical. They are afraid that if they fail, they will receive harsh criticism. They are afraid of rocking the boat when everything in their yearly reports indicates that they have been doing well. Or they are afraid that, if they begin to hold healing services and then are moved to another church, this may put a burden on the incoming spiritual leader. Above all, they are afraid to support healing because it is not part of the program of the church with which they are affiliated. Like Jesus, they could be seen as a threat to the very structure and power of the church if they fully followed His command to heal (and love).

Also, I said, pastors fear the criticism of the larger community. The negative publicity and negative influence of some spiritual healers makes the desirability of healing services in this or that respectable church seem questionable. And perhaps, behind all the other excuses, is a very human resistance to change. They are afraid to change when all seems to be going well in their ministries. They can imagine the burdens this would place upon them.

This part of my talk was not well received, though in the question-and-answer period that followed no challenges to my declarations were given directly.

One curious incident occurred during my address. A minister sitting near me was constantly rubbing his elbow and wincing. At one point I stopped my presentation and asked him if he would like to have me lay my hands on his elbow and pray. He was mightily embarrassed and declined. Several minutes passed. Then he interrupted me and came up to me. I prayed for his elbow and he was instantly healed. I did not understand why no other attender remarked about this healing.

UNENLIGHTENED CHURCH TEACHINGS

On another occasion I was led to write a newspaper article suggesting that the Christian church was unwittingly fostering an atmosphere in which cancer can grow more easily. The article was published.

The responses from the clergy were expected: "That's not true of my church," or "This sounds like blasphemy," and the like.

I was not surprised at the reception of the article. But I knew that putting out the message was important. I had grown heartsick at the virtual absence of any program for spiritual healing in the churches. It was clear to me that we have been told to go and teach, spread the Gospel, *and heal,* and that this directive should include today's age as well as the eras of the Old and New Testaments. Instead of support for healing, either through programs for spiritual healing or through emphasizing how to receive God's personal love, I was seeing what could be considered the exact opposite: The churches were teaching attitudes that contributed to illness.

I do not see any major change in churches today in terms of recognizing healers or fostering healing. My own denomination, the United Methodist Church, has sidestepped that command until very recently, when a prayer-for-healing service was incorporated into its approved rites, but there is no accommodation for recognizing a person—lay or clergy, male or female—who has been given the spiritual gift to heal. So I summarize the major points of the article here, to help people see that, whatever their church may be saying, God's miracles on behalf of humankind have not ceased.

The article dealt with the unwitting role of the church in fostering the advance of cancer and setting up blocks to its treatment, saying that the church did so by ten negative and destructive teachings. The article then pointed out what should be taught instead. Since much of what I said in that article is still true, I mention the main points here.

Innocently, the Christian church is providing an atmosphere in which cancer is attacking more and more people, I wrote, because the church is not encouraging basic attitudes within its devout for cancer to be avoided or, at least, treated successfully.

The public is being made abundantly aware, the article said, that some material substances are carcinogenic and that billions of dollars are being spent to find the "magic bullet" to kill cancer cells. Why was no such study being financed to study the *spiritual dimensions* of the cause and cure of cancer?

We know that cancer is characterized by the phenomenon of our own healthy cells double-crossing us and becoming predators, I continued. The discovery of some sort of inoculation to arrest this physical process is years ahead and possibly nonexistent. It seems reasonable to research what *other* factors contribute to this war within us, so we will be able to make adjustments to correct such destructive influences and bring a more holistic approach to the cure.

I know that cancer can be cured through spiritual healing, I wrote, for I have seen it happen before my very eyes. I have also observed that this healing process is often most difficult to heal when the ill persons have a background in the church and possess those prejudices we consider good qualities of the "faithful."

It is certainly true, I continued, that *all* the negative influences are not found in every person or that every branch of the Christian church is guilty in every instance. Still, the factors need to be listed.

The first negative factor impeding health that I have observed in church teaching is its overemphasis on guilt, I wrote.

We have long known that guilt (overt or hidden) causes mental and physical turmoil. But guilt is forgivable, and forgiveness and its ensuing state of inner peace is not something we earn; it is a free gift of God. Reconciliation of the individual with God prevents putrefaction.

So, I asked, why doesn't the church emphasize God's forgiveness? Emphasis upon God's judgment for sin—without the oft-cited scriptural reminders that God forgives—affects many persons who have not heard of this evidence of His caring for us and His forgiving love. The engendered fear is like a tumor growing within.

Second, the article continued, the church has, at least by omission, taught that illness is sometimes God's way of punishing us for our sins. It is only too easy to blame God when things go wrong. The church should be actively teaching that God never punishes anyone physically for anything. He retains the power of judgment, of course, but since the New Covenant, at least, illness has not been His weapon of retribution. God gave His Son to prove His love, and it is the church's job to teach a fuller understanding of the scope of His love.

Third, I wrote, the church has lamely declared that otherwise-unexplained tragedies are "God's will." This is more than a careless offering when spoken to a grieving family stricken with tragedy. This is blasphemy. God's will is always that everyone be happy and healthy.

Fourth, the church has taught people to be unselfish to an extreme, to always deny themselves and to always think of others first. The article pointed out that this overemphasis causes people problems when it comes to seeking healing. We cannot truly serve others until we are comfortably aware of our own value. There are times when a Christian must be *self*ish.

Fifth, the church has led people to believe that it is not right to complain when so many others are so much worse off than they are. My experience, I wrote, is that God does not heal only the most severe problems. Whatever is of concern to us is of concern to Him.

Sixth, the church has taught that we need to have FAITH (in capital letters), and that if we have enough of it, good things will happen to us, even healing. This is a convolution of how God works, I said, for I have seen unbelievers be healed. A full storehouse of faith is not, then, a prerequisite to healing, just as a person's *not* being healed is not a signal of a lack of his or her faith. God puts no price tag on His love.

Seventh, the church has led people to believe, by its treatment of the miracles recorded in the Scriptures as historical events of that day alone, that miracles are not likely to be evident in modern times. This is clearly not fact, the article said and I still say today. Though I'm approaching my eighties, I have never lost my excitement at the number of miracles I see almost daily. I can say from experience that dramatic, sudden, and complete cures are everyday events with God.

Eighth, while the church has convinced people that God is Love, it has failed to make it clear that His love is personal. I suggested that the church ask people to pray that favorite Scripture verse (John 3:16) this way: "God so loved *me* that He gave His only Son that whoever believes in Him should not perish but have everlasting life." God's love is most meaningful when it is personal.

Ninth, the church has taught people to be submissive to authority (the church, the Bible, the clergy, civil authorities), largely without question. When applied to healing, I wrote, this unquestioning submission tends to be extended to medical authorities. My experience is that we need to be an active partner in the healing process, not an inert lump of flesh.

Tenth, the church has taught that it is unseemly to express ourselves emotionally in rage, hurt, weeping, or joy. Both psychologically and spiritually speaking, I said, I have seen that pent-up emotions breed rebellion in our behavior and in our cellular structure.

I would still like to see more of these factors examined and de-emphasized in our churches. I believe that emphasizing the alternatives suggested in the preceding paraphrase of my newspaper article will bring changes in our communities on a scale that cannot easily be imagined.

• • •

In my work as an evangelist I have led services in many churches in New England. At the close of the service, after a message about the personal love of the God who seeks them out, I give the invitation for the people in the church to come to the altar. I tell them that the coming forward is not to confess their sins or receive forgiveness. It is not to ensure a seat in heaven, or to be saved as my Pentecostal brothers and sisters define salvation from eternal punishment. They are invited to come forward and kneel and just let God's love get through to them. It is an experience of receiving.

The altar area is always crowded. I have seen the joy in people's faces when they suddenly know their own worth.

There *is* joy. Do not ever forget:

> *Open the door and He will come in.*

Examples of Healing

There *are* still miracles in the world every day, not just scientific marvels, but works of God. In fact, miracles abound. We need only to expect them, recognize them when they happen, and praise God for them.

Is it so difficult to believe? Listen to what I have seen: Through my hands tumors disappear, the blind see, arthritic pain goes away, hearing is restored, persons in comas awaken, disfigured faces become clear, and much, much more. Like any spiritual healer, I know it is not I who possess the power to heal. God *is* still in the miracle business.

The experience of the laying on of hands is a humbling experience. I can feel that flow of power and it is as though power is leaving me. A wave of exhaustion follows a very "difficult" miracle. But I am quickly restored and move on to the next person.

While still a pastor in Spencer I continued to hold monthly healing services. Many were healed. Since I've retired, I still hold such services on non-church property, and healings are still being given by God through my hands. These services would not be possible without the strong support of my healing team. Elsie Harsha has been an especially strong supporter, serving as accompanist for the healing services since the beginning. Once, after a particularly tiring healing service I walked over to her and said, "What will I do when the line gets even longer?" She replied, "The Lord is with you and He will provide." She was right: He is and He does.

Another staunch supporter of the healing ministry from the early years at Spencer is Frank Hollows. Frank became the lay leader of the congregation. From the beginning of the healing ministry he has been the leader. I don't believe he has ever missed one of those services. He greets the people, makes announcements, and leads the singing of hymns. He also provides the soloists or other special music for the services. Then, while I'm ministering to the people in the healing line, he directs the congregation in more hymns or plays carefully selected tapes.

In addition to the healing services, I have seen many people, usually by appointment, in my office. There are so many more examples of healing that I could cite.

• • •

I remember Hans. His sister had been miraculously healed of scars on her face as the result of burns. This happened during a service I held for the Unification Church in Boston. She came through the line with little hope for any change. As

I prayed for healing and moved my fingers across those scars they smoothed out and disappeared. I stepped back to see her reaction. She didn't believe it until another girl in the line held up a pocket mirror. She fainted then, but quickly revived and ran about thanking God.

Hans phoned me from New York. He had come over from Germany after hearing of his sister's success, he said, and he had a bus ticket to Worcester and then out to Spencer. He gave me the approximate time of his arrival.

I waited for him at the church. Finally I heard him enter the door just down the steps from my office. He came into the church and I could see him standing there, held up by two crutches. I went to the head of the flight of stairs, six of them, and simply said, "Come on up, Hans. Leave your crutches there."

He hesitated only a few seconds and then came steadily up those steps. I waved him into an adjoining hall, and he went in there and began walking and then running around the room. We had lunch together and I got him on the bus for his return trip.

He wrote me a week later and said he would never again need the crutches he had left on the floor.

• • •

In His farewell conversations with His disciples, Jesus referred to the things they had heard from Him and the miracles He had performed. Then He said (in John 14:12), "I tell you the truth, anyone who has faith in Me will do what I have been doing. He will do even greater things than these, for I am going to my Father." That has always bothered me. I am not Christ and I stand in awe of the great miracles He performed. For me to do *greater* things is beyond my imagination. But I have never failed to meet the challenge of someone facing me for healing.

That does not mean that I never experience a feeling of inadequacy. Just before one of my healing services began in Spencer, some people rolled in a gurney with an eighteen-year-old lad lying on it. They had put him in front of the pews. I glanced down at him frequently during the early part of the service. Eventually I went down to him. He was the only survivor of an auto accident. He had received numerous injuries: skull fracture, both legs broken, his eyesight and hearing gone. He could not talk but he keened aloud! Where should I start? I had to ask God. He answered.

I prayed and touched Jimmy's ears and he heard. His moaning stopped. I touched his eyes and he saw. I touched his mouth and he spoke, hesitatingly at first and then with more assurance. The people in the congregation were excited and began to shout praise and thanks to God.

After that day I visited him at his home, and after six months his restoration was complete. He stood, he walked, he talked, he was joyful. I lost touch with the family after I moved away and he graduated from high school.

• • •

A couple with their nine-year-old daughter were on their way to a vacation on Nantucket when the child was stricken so ill that they took her to Children's Hospital in Boston. She was found to have leukemia The grandmother, who lived in my town, phoned and asked me to visit her.

After driving to the hospital with the grandmother, I took the little girl in my arms and prayed for healing. We then went to a visitors' room to talk. Shortly after, the nurse came in to tell us that another blood test had been taken. We waited for the results: No trace of leukemia could be found.

The next day the child went to Nantucket with her parents. They phoned me a year later to tell me that she had had no recurrence.

• • •

A lady was diagnosed with a malignant cancer in her uterus. I laid hands on her for healing. She underwent a hysterectomy.

The doctor sent me a letter saying, "Following the operation the pathology reported a necrotic (dead) tumor with no viable residual mixed mesodermal tumor."

• • •

A young woman lost the sight of her left eye. It was instantly restored during a service.

• • •

My dental hygienist, after she had cleaned my teeth, asked me to heal her lupus. As I prayed, she felt tremors throughout her body. Three days later she phoned and then wrote me to say that she had been healed.

She had not been going to church, but after her healing both she and her family resumed going to church.

• • •

An aneurysm behind a woman's lung created unbearable pain. When I held my hand on her chest, the pain left. In the emergency room I prayed with her.

The next CAT scan showed no sign of the mass of blood.

• • •

I have a photograph of a little girl eating an ice cream cone. She had that treat on her way home after being healed of lactose intolerance.

• • •

A young man, a victim of an auto accident, was in a coma for three months. He was swathed in bandages. I laid my hands on his head and called him to awaken.

He sat up in bed and asked for a drink of milk and greeted his mother.

• • •

The call came early one morning. It was a young man from New York, and he told me he had heard of my healing ministry and asked if I could help him. I promised him I'd try. Then he said, "I'm Jewish. Does that make a difference?" I assured him it did not—after all, Jesus was a Jew. So he made arrangements.

His daughter was in a Jewish hospital on Long Island. They wanted to send me plane tickets there and back to Hartford. His little girl, twelve years old, had leukemia. She was in a light coma. The doctors had little hope for her.

They met me at the airport and we drove to the hospital. I found Becky in a room on a floor filled with children with all kinds of cancer, all of them regarded as terminal. Becky was being fed intravenously. She did not open her eyes, but squeezed her mother's hand. She was little more than a skeleton. A pathetic sight.

I held her hand and prayed briefly for her and walked out of the room. I found a place where I could be alone and there I brought my petition to God. "You helped the daughter of Jairus when everyone thought she was dead. I need to restore this little child."

I went back into the room and leaned over the sleeping figure. I raised her up and held her and prayed for a miracle. In a few moments she began to stir and then sat up. I moved back and her mother took my place. Becky spoke. "Could I have a milk shake?" she asked. The nurse was called in. Needless to say there was great joy in that room.

A week later Becky's father called me and said that Becky was home and recovering her strength. Three years later the three of them came by my church and we had a joyous reunion.

•••

A dear lady, eighty-two years of age, stunned a congregation when she received her sight, which she had lost when a child.

•••

Have I been asked to heal animals? Yes, they are God's creatures too. Once one of the church ladies came unannounced into my office with her pet. She told me that she was worried about it and would I pray for healing? I would, and I bent down to the basket.

In it was what I took to be a big fat cat. I petted the animal but neglected to ask what the trouble was. I asked God for healing.

The woman took her pet home and called me the next day to say her pet was okay again. A few days later I saw her and asked how her cat was. She stiffened slightly and sharply corrected me, saying, "It is a bunny."

Healers are not always right!

•••

Members of a family from Ashland, Massachusetts, became my clients. It began with Gail, a young business executive who had suffered a brain aneurysm. I first met her in church after her surgery. She was still heavily medicated with phenobarbital and unable to work. She acted lackadaisical and slow. Her first introduction to me had been while listening to one of my sermons and she hadn't liked it at all. But she had continued to come to my church, had learned of my healing ministry, and now came seeking a miracle.

The healing was instantaneous. She was most grateful. At her next visit to her doctor, he declared her fully healed and took her off the drugs.

Gail had been traumatized by the ordeal, though, and continued to see me each week for a while, for reinforcement. In a little while she met and fell in love with a fine young man, and they determined to get married. Gail went to her doctor to get his reassurance and approval to marry. He gave it, and I performed the ceremony.

In a few months they wanted to start a family. Again the doctor told them there was no reason she should fear pregnancy since she was well and had been off all medication for some time. They had a healthy baby boy, and I baptized him. Since then they have had another son and all is well with them.

At one point in my association with Gail, her father became crippled in the left leg with arthritis. At her request, I went to their home and laid my hands on his knee. He stood up, the pain gone.

Weeks after that, her mother was diagnosed with breast cancer. She came to one of my public healing services and asked for a miracle. She was healed. Five years later she is still cancer free.

Afterword

It happened while Jesus was walking along the road on the way to another healing mission. The crowd pressed about Him, asking for His favors. He stopped momentarily. A woman made her way up to Him and crouched at His feet. This story is told in the ninth chapter of Matthew. The woman had said to herself, "If I could but touch the hem of His garment I could be healed." Jesus felt this movement at His feet and asked who had touched Him. "How can we tell?" the disciples answered. "There are so many here." Then the Lord noticed the woman and said to her, "Take heart, daughter, your faith has made you whole." And she was healed through touching the hem of His garment! She put out her shaking hands and touched, and the touch healed her.

The Lord still makes His way along the roads today with His love and His healing power. We cannot hear His human voice. We cannot see the scars in his hands. His robe is long gone. But the hem of his garment is still here. An old hymn ("Dear Lord and Father of Mankind") expresses the thought for us: "The healing of His seamless dress is by our beds of pain; We touch Him in life's throng and press, and we are whole again."

The healing hem of His garment is indeed still among us. I want to continue to be one who offers that healing touch to others. I encourage you to use your gifts for God also.

APPENDIX

Some Theological Thoughts

Remind everyone of these things, and command them in God's name to stop fighting over words. Such arguments are useless, and they can ruin those who hear them.

—2 Timothy 2:14 NLV

The Holy Spirit

The Holy Spirit is God within us. Jesus called Him the Comforter. He told His disciples He was going away but would not leave them comfortless. He said, in His farewell conversations with His disciples, "I will ask the Father, and He will give you another Comforter to be with you forever, the Spirit of Truth" (John 14:16–17). Jesus continued, "All this have I spoken while still with you. But the Comforter, the Holy Spirit, whom the Father will send in My name, will teach you all things and will remind you of everything I have said to you" (John 14:25–26). Jesus then told the disciples to wait, and the Holy Spirit would come upon them.

The story of the coming of the Holy Spirit is told in the dramatic events described in the second chapter of Acts. With the power of the Spirit the disciples went forward to preach the word of the kingdom. The Holy Spirit is in anyone who allows that Spirit to be a part of his or her inner life. The Spirit exists as conscience, as a guide, as empowerment. It is important to realize that this was part of God's plan for revelation: the culmination of His relationship with mankind. After the days of the hero figures of the Old Testament—of kings and champions, of the prophets (each of whom added to the understanding of what God is like and what His will is)—and after the coming of Jesus, the Holy Spirit was made available as God within us. Each person possesses the immense potential of working with that Spirit in the course of his or her life.

It should be noted that the Holy Spirit was not available to everyone in this way in the Old Testament. It is true that the Spirit of God entered the life of a particular chosen person to perform some great task, but He was available only to a few anointed ones.

The potential presence of the Holy Spirit within the life of each person today should make everyone all the more important in our sight. No matter how degraded one may become, he or she is redeemable and must be approached as such. I see the application of this great truth as an important factor in the practice of spiritual healing.

Prayer

The apostle Paul once wrote, "Pray without ceasing." We must know that he wasn't referring to the person who, asked to "say grace" at table, keeps intoning pious mutterings while the steaks grow cold. I believe he meant that prayer ought to be a way of living. I remember E. Stanley Jones saying one time, "Sometimes I am so tired when I go to bed that I don't feel up to saying my prayers. So I simply say, 'Lord, you remember my prayer of last night. Hear it again for me.' " We will not be heard because of the length of our speaking. *Life* ought to be a prayer so that we communicate with God wherever we are: not necessarily in a church, kneeling with our eyes closed. We can be driving our cars, working that machine, looking up at the sky. *Whatever* we are doing, God is at our elbow and He hears us. The Spirit is within us believers and we are one with that Spirit.

Once, at my first meeting with the United Methodist Women at a church where I had recently arrived as pastor, I listened to a long discussion of business matters, which seemed necessary. The hour grew late and I was tired. Someone finally turned to me and said, "Pastor, will you give us a prayer and maybe an address?" I replied, "I'll give you a prayer and it will be a benediction. As far as my address goes, let it be the same as your last pastor's."

Don't misunderstand me, please. I love to pray and listen to the prayers of others. Only when praying becomes mechanical, done because it's the thing to do, do I grow restless.

Sin

My definition of sin is similar to my thoughts about prayer. Sin is not so much the committing of an evil act or thinking evil thoughts, it is a turning away from God the Holy Spirit. When we reject the Spirit at any particular moment in our lives, we become separated from the Spirit's guidance and thus open to sinful urges. That very state of separation is sin.

Frantic Fatalists vs. Kingdom Builders

Apocalypse is a word that is often spoken in the same way as someone calling out, "Dial 911!" at the time of an accident. It's somewhat scary. Apocalyptic material deals with the predictions as to what will happen to this earth in "the last days." Jonathan Edwards, pioneer preacher in New England in the 1800s, had a wide reputation for making it clear what would happen to us when the world comes to an end: A few would be saved and the rest thrown into an everlasting flame. It is said that Jonathan Edwards was so graphic in his warnings and his descriptions of hell that, in response, strong men clung to the pews in front of them and women fainted.

Some sects today are convinced that their way is right and the rest of us are doomed. They will appear at your door and try to save you. I remember a group of them who came to Martha's Vineyard while I was there and caused disturbance among the churchpeople of Vineyard Haven. Our church's congregation did not want to be impolite but they also did not want to spend time listening to this version of Christianity.

They asked me what to do when the group came knocking. One of our ladies offered a solution.

She told us that, when two well-dressed young women came to her door, she opened it and greeted them. Before they could say more she asked them if they had come to discuss religion. They admitted they had. So she swung the door wide open and said, "Great, come in! Let's take our clothes off and talk about it! I'm a nudist!" They retreated.

The religionists who believe that we are all born damned, and must spend our lives earning our way upward, speak of a cataclysmic act by a vengeful God whose patience has reached an end and decides on a Day of Judgment to separate the good from the bad. The good will be swept into heaven and the evil cast into hell. No one knows when this awful event will take place, but every now and then some fiery-eyed prophet of doom will predict a day. There is a tiny flurry of activity, sometimes characterized by people selling off all their goods and retreating to a mountaintop so that their trip to heaven will be shorter.

The whole Christian scene, then, can be divided into two groups. These groups are not named as such, but I like to call them the "kingdom builders" and the "frantic fatalists."

The kingdom builders believe that God will never give up on us and on the noble experiment of God and man working together to bring heaven on earth. They cannot see the possibility of failure. They take to heart the line in the Lord's Prayer that says, "Thy kingdom come . . . on earth as it is in heaven." The kingdom builders are motivated by the order of Jesus to go into all the world and preach the kingdom.

The frantic fatalists try to change society too, but they do so with the security of knowing that *they* will be among the ones who will be saved. It seems to me that this belief robs them of some of their fervor in evangelizing. For they are essentially saying, "I'll warn you and I'll try to save you, but if you don't heed my message you will have to take the consequences." The frantic fatalists believe that a war is being waged between God and a "fallen angel," Satan.

I am a kingdom builder, and I am still excited daily at what God will do right here on earth, whenever we allow Him to work through us.

Satan

Flip Wilson used to say, "The devil made me do it!"

The belief in the person of Satan was and is an attempt to blame our evil actions on a convenient theological concept. The thesis is preserved by eliciting fear of that supposedly powerful force, and solicitation of sympathy from a God who is aware of mankind's dilemma.

Jonathan Edwards thundered from the pulpit to scare the hell out of people. He has some imitators today!

Scripture references to Satan depict incidents attributed to him and reach primitive conclusions typical of ages before the enlightenment of science.

But if God is the Supreme Being of all existence how could He have a rival?

If heaven is truly Paradise as described in Scripture, no possibility is provided for the existence of an evil angel!

There are wayward tendencies in us all. We gain this unwholesome heritage by exposure to a host of people, beginning with (with no evil intent) our own family.

Flip Wilson was wrong: There is no devil! Sorry, people.

Sermonizing

There are two basic methods of finding themes for clergy to use as sermon subjects. The Roman Catholic Church and the mainline Protestant denominations (for the most part) follow the lectionary, one basic method of finding a theme to preach about. The lectionary is a selected list of Scripture readings for every day of the year. It is prepared, I believe, three years in advance. I haven't been able to discover what the source is, but the scholarship is of top quality. The minister who uses the lectionary has three Bible readings each Sunday: one from the Old Testament, one from the letters of Paul (or others), and one from the Gospels. The three readings are tied together, showing similarity in themes.

The advantages of using the lectionary are obvious: It provides continuity across the year, makes it obvious that the messages of the various books of the Bible are intertwined, and provides discipline and scholarship in the use of God's book. Other advantages are not as obvious, but they include knowing what you're going to preach about on any given Sunday so that you can prepare ahead, and making certain that you diversify your themes. With the lectionary method, there are many companion books available that list suggested hymns, prayers, and responsive readings. In addition, other scholars have provided books of sermons on just those same subjects on those same passages.

There is a problem with the lectionary method, and that problem is why I am not fond of the lectionary. When I think of this method, I cannot help asking, Where does the Holy Spirit play a role in the inspiration needed to provide relevant messages to our congregations? Does the Holy Spirit only go to work at those meetings where the lectionary is devised? Does this method have a tendency to make people who give homilies lazy? Are they in touch weekly with the current needs of the persons in their church's pews? These are questions we dare not avoid. The Holy Spirit is not needed only in healing. The Holy Spirit is needed in the matter of sermonizing too.

The other basic method is the exposition of Scripture—the method used by most clergy. In this method a scriptural passage (or more than one) is lifted up. To prepare the sermon the sermonizer may refer to commentaries, Bible dictionaries, hundreds of books of sermons on related subjects—a seemingly unending source of material. In this method the text is the root of the message, and much attention is given to it. For many years the churchpeople have applauded this style of preaching. They are fond of saying, "That's preaching from the Word!"

Like the lectionary method, this method of finding themes for sermon subjects relies upon the use of the Word of God. In this method, however, the preacher is filled with the desire to bring that Word to the people who have shown a need for a particular subject. The pastor in touch with his or her flock has no problem finding something needful to bring. But the relevant *topic* is the focus of the discourse: Scripture is used to enforce, to illustrate, to declare what is the most plausible will of the Creator in a given circumstance.

One Spiritual Adventure Group

The guiding principle of our Adventure Groups' perusal of selected Bible passages is to accept the inspiration as fact and then boldly claim that God is still in the business of inspiration. We look at a passage together, without the instructions about the time and circumstances deemed necessary by the usual methods of adult Bible study, and ask God to inspire our reading, our thinking, and our offering of those insights to other members of the group. We then close the Book and talk about what we remember about the passage.

This method takes practice because most new participants have been well trained to expect the teacher to teach them! Once they get used to the idea that there is no teacher in this group and so they might do better to forgo their comments about extraneous details, the Spirit within them goes to work. Their potential to be inspired comes forth, and they offer insights to the group. Each offering is applauded, without judgment, by the group. As they get used to the thrill of receiving inspiration, the offerings of the group members become more exciting, and even priceless!

During one Christian season of Lent, I was assigned a portion of Scripture to use as my text when it came my turn to preach as part of the forty-day journey through the events of the passion of Jesus. My text was to be Mark 15:1–15.

I don't like preaching from assigned texts but I could see the purpose of this series, so I took the story to a Christian Adventure Group and asked them to help me find a sermon in it.

They fell to work. That passage tells the story of Jesus being brought before Pilate and the accusations made against Him:

> *The religious leaders of the day are demanding His death. Pilate, the Roman governor of that region, has little respect for the Jewish leaders and tries to avoid appeasing them by pronouncing the desired death sentence.*
>
> *Someone reminds him that, at that particular season, it is the custom to release some criminal who will soon be put to death. So Pilate offers the Jewish people the choice: Jesus or Barabbas. Barabbas was a guerilla fighter who had a record of leading incursions against small bands of Roman soldiers and who had been found guilty of killing a number of them. The contrast with Jesus is obvious.*
>
> *But the scribes and Pharisees stir up the people by strategically placing among the crowd their henchmen, who call out for the release of Barabbas. The people follow the henchmen's lead and call for the crucifixion of Jesus.*

> *Jesus does not defend Himself before Pilate but remains silent. Pilate releases Barabbas, has Jesus flogged, and orders His execution.*

I asked the Christian Adventure Group how this story could be used to show a truth far greater than that in the details already found in the story.

The group wrestled with the problem, asking questions like: Can we imagine a similar situation today? In what way can we bring out a challenge from this story? What important truth from this story should live on?

Bits and pieces were put together. It was a joyful experience to see the inspiration at work. No one offering was enough: The group worked together, adding first one idea, then another until the effort was rewarded.

It was decided that the story's real impact could be found in the love for mankind portrayed in that dramatic confrontation: Jesus did not defend Himself (He knew that His fate was preordained, that He was to pay for the sins of the world). The contrast of the figure of Pilate standing above Jesus underscored the majesty and righteousness of the Accused. His humiliation was part of His sacrificial offering. Being flogged was part of the price for our sins that Jesus accepted for Himself. How moving is the picture of Jesus submitting to this degradation as a further indication of how *much* He loves us!

How is this theme relevant today?

Another group may find in this passage some completely different applications to their situation. This group answered the question this way: God still labors to let us know how important we are to Him, how vast His love for us is. Having submitted to Pilate, what more does Jesus have to do to convince us today? Here I had an opportunity to share my thought by reminding the class, and later my congregation, of the leading obstacle to people's believing that God will work the miracle of healing for them: the difficulty of truly believing that He loves them personally.

For now we see in a mirror, dimly, but then we will see face to face. Now I know only in part; then I will know fully, even as I have been fully known. And now faith, hope, and love abide, these three; and the greatest of these is love.
　　　　　　　　　　　—1 Corinthians 13:12–13 NRSV